CUTANEOUS T-CELL LYMPHOMA

Mycosis Fungoides and
Sezary Syndrome

CUTANEOUS T-CELL LYMPHOMA

Mycosis Fungoides and Sezary Syndrome

Edited by

Herschel S. Zackheim, M.D.
Department of Dermatology
University of California, San Francisco

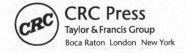

CRC Press
Taylor & Francis Group
Boca Raton London New York

CRC Press
Taylor & Francis Group
6000 Broken Sound Parkway NW, Suite 300
Boca Raton, FL 33487-2742

First issued in paperback 2019

ISBN-13: 978-0-8493-2101-6 (hbk)
ISBN-13: 978-0-367-39367-0 (pbk)

Library of Congress Card Number 2004054469

Library of Congress Cataloging-in-Publication Data
Cutaneous T-cell lymphoma : mycosis fungoides and Sézary syndrome / edited by Herschel S. Zackheim.
p.   cm. — (Dermatology : clinical & basic science series)
Includes bibliographical references and index.
ISBN 0-8493-2101-8 (alk. paper)
1. Mycosis fungoides. 2. Lymphomas. 3. Skin—umors. I. Zackheim, Herschel S. II. Dermatology (CRC Press)
[DNLM: 1. Lymphoma, T-Cell, Cutaneous. WH 525 C9887 204]
RC280.L9C873 2004
616.99′477de 22   2004054469

Series Preface

Our goal in creating the *Dermatology: Clinical & Basic Science Series* is to present the insights of experts on emerging applied and experimental techniques and theoretical concepts that are, or will be, at the vanguard of dermatology. These books cover new and exciting multidisciplinary areas of cutaneous research, and we want them to be the books every physician will use to become acquainted with new methodologies in skin research. These books can be also given to graduate students and postdoctoral fellows when they are looking for guidance to start a new line of research.

The series consists of books that are edited by experts, with chapters written by the leaders in each particular field. The books are richly illustrated and contain comprehensive bibliographies. Each chapter provides substantial background material relevant to its subject. These books contain detailed tricks of the trade and information regarding where the methods presented can be safely applied. In addition, information on where to buy equipment and helpful Web sites for solving both practical and theoretical problems are included.

We are working with these goals in mind. As the books become available, the efforts of the publisher, book editors, and individual authors will contribute to the further development of dermatology research and clinical practice. The extent to which we achieve this goal will be determined by the utility of these books.

Howard I. Maibach, M.D.

Preface

Although cutaneous T-cell lymphoma (CTCL) is relatively rare, it is of considerable interest to dermatologists as well as oncologists. One of the prime reasons for this is that CTCL is one of a relatively small number of dermatoses that has the potential for a fatal outcome. Particularly in its early stage, CTCL is often difficult to diagnose, both clinically and histologically. Further, CTCL has many forms of clinical presentations that may mimic other dermatoses.

The present volume presents an overview of the epidemiology and salient clinical and histologic features of mycosis fungoides, the most common form of CTCL. Related forms of CTCL, including Sezary syndrome, lymphomatoid papulosis, cutaneous CD30+ anaplastic large cell lymphoma, and follicular mucinosis, are reviewed. Immunochemistry and molecular techniques for diagnosis, as well as molecular abnormalities, are discussed. The volume concludes with a survey of the state-of-the-art treatment of CTCL and a section on staging and prognosis.

Editor

Herschel S. Zackheim is clinical professor of dermatology at the University of California, San Francisco (UCSF) and has been director of the Cutaneous Lymphoma Clinic there since 1973. He received his B.A. at New York University in 1937 and his M.D. at the University of Michigan in 1942.

He is the author or co-author of more than 140 peer-reviewed publications, mostly concerning cutaneous lymphomas. He is a member of the International Society for Cutaneous Lymphomas, San Francisco Dermatological Society, and other dermatological societies. His honors include Dermatology Foundation Practitioner of the Year, 1986; Special Recognition Award, Association of the Clinical Faculty, UCSF, 1996; Practitioner of the Year, San Francisco Dermatology Society, 2000; Honorary Member, American Academy of Dermatology, 2001; Certificate of Appreciation, International League of Dermatological Societies, 2004.

Contributors

Lawrence E. Gibson, M.D.
Department of Dermatology
Mayo Clinic
Mayo Foundation
Rochester, Minnesota

H.L. Greenberg, M.D.
Department of Dermatology
University of Wisconsin
Madison, Wisconsin
and
Middleton Veterans Affairs Medical
  Center
Madison, Wisconsin

Mohammed Kashani-Sabet, M.D.
Department of Dermatology
University of California, San Francisco
San Francisco, California

**Maria M. Morales Suárez-Varela,
M.D., Ph.D.**
Unit of Public Health and
  Environmental Care
Department of Preventive Medicine and
  Public Health
Valencia University
and
Unit of Clinical Epidemiology
University Hospital
Dr. Peset
Valencia, Spain

Bruce R. Smoller, M.D.
University of Arkansas for Medical
  Sciences
Little Rock, Arkansas

Sean Whittaker, M.D., F.R.C.P.
St John's Institute of Dermatology
Guy's and St Thomas' Hospital
London, England
and
Department Division of Skin Sciences
King's College London
London, England

Anne E. Wilkerson, M.D.
University of Arkansas for Medical
  Sciences
Little Rock, Arkansas

Gary S. Wood, M.D.
Department of Dermatology
University of Wisconsin
Madison, Wisconsin
and
Middleton Veterans Affairs Medical
  Center
Madison, Wisconsin

Herschel S. Zackheim, M.D.
Department of Dermatology
University of California, San Francisco
San Francisco, California

Contents

1 Mycosis Fungoides: Epidemiology

Maria M. Morales Suárez-Varela

CONTENTS

1.1 INTRODUCTION

Mycosis fungoide (MF) cases make up the great majority (80%–85%) of cases of primary cutaneous T-cell lymphoma (CTCL). CTCL is a lymphoproliferative disorder of epidermotropic, neoplastic T cells with a wide range of clinical manifestations. A number of other cutaneous disorders may present as different clinical manifestations of MF.[1]

MF was first described by Alibert et al.[2] in 1806. In 1876, Bazin et al.[3] defined the three stages of the disease (patches, plaques, and tumors).

The term CTCL was introduced by Lutzner et al.[4] in 1975 to describe a group of malignant lymphomas with primary manifestations in the skin. All forms of CTCL are neoplasms of T lymphocytes, which home to the skin and to the T-cell zones of lymphoid structures, but generally not to bone marrow. General lymphoma pathologists had different classifications of lymphoma, only one of which includes cutaneous lymphoma, as was first introduced by the Kiel classification in 1980 and updated in 1988.[5] Unfortunately, this classification is of limited value for those involved with cutaneous lymphoma because it is based on a detailed pathological assessment with no clinical correlation.

The two main classification systems used for cutaneous lymphomas are the Revised European-American Lymphoma (REAL) classification[6] and the system created by the European Organization for Research and Treatment of Cancer (EORTC).[7] Both schemata refine and extend older systems such as the Working Formulation[8] because they are based on a combination of clinicopathological, immunophenotypical, and molecular biological characteristics.

1.2 INCIDENCE

The reported standardized incidence rates for CTCL — of which MF is a subgroup — vary considerably. CTCL is an uncommon neoplasm, and the Surveillance, Epidemiology, and End Results program[9] reports that the incidence had increased 3.2-fold between 1973 and 1984, from 0.19 cases to 0.42 cases per 100,000 (Table 1.1). The overall incidence rate is approximately 4 to 5 per 1,000,000, according to data from that particular program,[10] where this tendency is seen in all the age, race, and sex groups (Tables 1.2, 1.3, 1.4, and 1.5).[9] In this time period 721 new cases were diagnosed, and a mean incidence was seen of 0.29 per 100,000 per year in the United States (probably due to an improvement in the diagnosis), which represented 2.2% of all lymphomas.[9,11]

TABLE 1.1

Incidence of Mycosis Fungoides and the Total of Lymphomas

	Mycosis Fungoides		Total Lymphomas	
Year	No. of Cases per 100,000 Inhabitants per Year	No. of Cases	No. of Cases per 100,000 Inhabitants per Year	No. of Cases
1973	0.19	30	11.69	1898
1974	0.17	32	11.93	2255
1975	0.23	47	12.18	2505
1976	0.19	39	11.97	2485
1977	0.30	63	12.05	2562
1978	0.25	52	12.51	2700
1979	0.28	60	13.01	2846
1980	0.23	53	12.87	2878
1981	0.34	77	13.66	3097
1982	0.36	83	13.71	3151
1983	0.38	88	14.07	3283
1984	0.42	97	14.79	3498

Note: Data are from the Surveillance, Epidemiology, and End Results Program.

Source: Weinstock, M.A. and Horm, J.W. *JAMA* 60, 42, 1988. With permission.

TABLE 1.2

Age When the Diagnosis Was Made in a Case Series According to Race and Sex

Age (Years)	Number (%) of Mycosis Fungoides Cases				
	White Men	White Women	Nonwhite Men	Nonwhite Women	Total
25–29	4 (3.4)	2 (3.2)	0	1 (7.1)	7 (3.3)
30–34	2 (1.7)	0	2 (11.8)	1 (7.1)	5 (2.4)
35–39	3 (2.5)	4 (6.5)	1 (5.9)	1 (7.1)	9 (4.3)
40–44	9 (7.6)	7 (11.3)	0	2 (14.3)	18 (8.5)
45–49	24 (20.3)	8 (12.9)	2 (11.8)	0	34 (16.1)
50–54	15 (12.7)	10 (16.1)	5 (29.4)	2 (14.3)	32 (15.2)
55–59	10 (8.5)	6 (9.7)	1 (5.9)	4 (28.6)	21 (10.0)
60–64	13 (11.0)	9 (14.5)	2 (11.8)	1 (7.1)	25 (11.8)
65–69	14 (11.9)	4 (6.5)	4 (23.5)	1 (7.1)	23 (10.9)
70–74	11 (9.3)	6 (9.7)	0	0	18 (8.5)
75–79	5 (4.2)	4 (6.5)	0	0	9 (4.3)
80–84	4 (3.4)	0	0	0	4 (1.9)
85–89	1 (0.8)	1 (1.6)	0	0	2 (1.0)
Unknown	3 (2.5)	1 (1.6)	0	0	4 (1.9)
Total	118	62	17	14	211

Source: From Greene, M.H. et al. *Cancer Treat. Rep.* 63, 597, 1979. With permission.

A similar tendency was seen in different European studies.[12,13] In Denmark, the MF incidence rate in 1987 was 0.2 per 100,000 in men, whereas only one case in 2.6 million was diagnosed in women.[12]

In a North American study,[9] the association that existed between the incidence of the disease and the concentration of doctors in each studied area suggests the bias in the detection of cases could be explained by differences in the geographical distribution, as those areas with a greater number of physicians showed a greater incidence level, possibly more consistent with earlier diagnosis. A 3.2-fold increase was described in the incidence of MF during the course of the study, and the proportion of MF cases among lymphomas increased from 1.6% to 2.8% over the course of the study.

The present-day incidence rate may be of a higher magnitude,[9] given the possible under-reporting and both the difficulty and confusion in making the diagnosis. The incidence of CTCL rises with age and is approximately twice (2.2 times) as common in men as in women, while blacks have twice the incidence of whites (Table 1.2).

Although CTCL cases in general, and MF cases in particular, are rarely seen before the age of 30,[14] they have been identified in children and teenagers.[15–18] However, the mean age at onset is 50 years.[19,20] Greene et al.[19] observed that the illness predominates in men (85%), generally middle-aged men (64% were found to be between 45 and 69 years of age). Table 1.2 shows the distribution of 211 MF cases with regard to age, race, and sex according to an American study carried out between 1950 and 1975 (excluding 1972).[19] According to the data obtained in the county of Los Angeles between 1972 and 1985, a greater incidence continues to be seen among the black race, where the ratio between the sexes is near to one (similar to the ratio in the white race).[21]

The data belonging to Third World countries are particularly scarce; in fact, most of the incidence data are limited to developed countries, especially the United States and European countries. However, MF appears to represent a lesser ratio of NHL in China (0.4%)[22] than in the United States (2.2% of all the lymphomas determined between the years 1973 and 1984).[23]

The gradual increase of incidence with age is presented in all the race and sex strata (Table 1.3).[9]

TABLE 1.3

Incidence of Mycosis Fungoides and the Total of Lymphomas According to Age, Race, and Sex

	Mycosis Fungoides		Total Lymphoma	
	No. of Cases per 100,000 Inhabitants per Year	No. of Cases	No. of Cases per 100,000 Inhabitants per Year	No. of Cases
Age (Years)				
< 40	0.05	90	4.08	7312
40–49	0.34	88	10.94	2830
50–59	0.56	143	21.05	5378
60–69	0.98	190	37.55	7264
70–79	1.28	144	59.72	6744
≥ 80	1.26	66	67.80	3627
Race				
Whites				
Total	0.26	568	13.46	29.977
Men	0.37	367	15.77	15.711
Women	0.17	201	11.56	14.266
Blacks				
Total	0.52	98	8.73	1742
Men	0.75	61	11.15	1016
Women	0.33	37	6.71	726
All races				
Total	0.29	721	12.95	33.155
Men	0.41	466	15.25	17.559
Women	0.19	255	11.03	15.596

Note: Data correspond to the years 1973–1984 from the Surveillance, Epidemiology, and End Results Program.

Source: Data from Weinstock, M.A. and Horm, J.W. *JAMA* 60, 42, 1988. With permission.

During the period 1979 to 1992, Weinstock et al.[24] described an incidence rate in the United States of 0.36/10 person-years;[25] there was no evidence of increasing incidence rates during the period 1983 through 1992, but the disorder varies greatly among demographic and geographic subgroups (Tables 1.4 and 1.5).

1.3 ETIOLOGY

Although the etiology of MF is unknown, Rowden and Lewis[29] posed the hypothesis that MF may begin to develop as a result of a primary alteration in cellular immune response, mediated by the Langerhans cells. The suspicion that a persistent antigenic stimulation could play an important role in MF development was suggested for the first time by Tan et al.[30] in 1974, based on the findings of high IgE levels in patients affected by MF.

Several causative factors have been proposed and subsequently investigated. These include chronic antigenic stimulation as a result of different exposures to bacterial infections, smoking, medications, chronic sun exposure, viral infections, and chemical exposition.

The marked variation of MF incidence through time and the absence of a documented family association suggest that MF is not a primary genetic disorder, although that does not imply that it does not present a certain grade of genetic predisposition. Also, the association of MF with a family history of Hodgkin's disease has been documented, although the presence of certain potential factors (environmental or hereditary) has not been determined.[31]

In a study carried out in the United States on 211 patients affected by MF, 26% (56 patients) were noted to have a close family member who also presented some type of skin disease. Thirty percent (63 patients) had a close family member with a history of cancer. And 20% (42 patients) had some close family member who was affected by cancer.[19]

Between December 1976 and February 1977 Cohen et al.[32] studied family cancer medical histories by means of an interview in which the following data were included: job name, production, activity, the usual work one was assigned to, and a description of its activity. A family medical history was considered as positive if any member who was genetically related to the family was diagnosed with cancer, no matter which type; the finding of a family cancer medical history in both the cases studied and the control subjects had a similar frequency. The probability of finding a positive family medical history of cancer among the study patients was similar to 1 (RR = 1.1).

In the California/Washington study,[32] a significant association was noted between MF and a history of other malignant diseases different than non-Hodgkin lymphoma or skin cancer (RR = 3.3, p <.001), probably due to the Berkson bias (this bias deals with the possible existence of spurious associations between different diseases, or between a disease and a risk factor).[33] A more extensive and subsequent study performed with data from the Cancer Register in the United States showed the absence of an association between MF and previous malignant diseases and suggests that certain aspects of the California/Washington study could have led to

TABLE 1.4

Incidence of Mycosis Fungoides, Specifically by Age, Race, and Sex in Selected Areas

Age	White Men		White Women		Black Men		Black Women	
	No. of Cases per 100,000 Inhabitants per Year	No. of Cases	No. of Cases per 100,000 Inhabitants per Year	No. of Cases	No. of Cases per 100,000 Inhabitants per Year	No. of Cases	No. of Cases per 100,000 Inhabitants per Year	No. of Cases
< 50	0.10	79	0.05	42	0.23	17	0.20	20
50–59	0.69	74	0.32	36	1.61	15	0.47	5
60–69	1.35	106	0.57	52	2.82	18	0.64	5
≥ 70	1.92	108	0.77	71	2.97	11	1.28	7

Note: Data are from the Surveillance, Epidemiology, and End Results Program.

Source: Weinstock, M.A. and Horm, J.W. *JAMA* 60, 42, 1988. With permission.

TABLE 1.5
Incidence of Mycosis Fungoides Adjusted to Age, According to the Year of Diagnosis, Race, Sex, Age and Registration Date in Selected Areas of the United States

	1973–1976		1977–1980		1981–1984	
	No. of Cases per 100,000 Inhabitants per Year	No. of Cases	No. of Cases per 100,000 Inhabitants per Year	No. of Cases	No. of Cases per 100,000 Inhabitants per Year	No. of Cases
Race and Sex						
White men	0.28	83	0.34	116	0.47	168
White women	0.11	42	0.15	63	0.23	96
Black men	0.49	12	0.78	22	0.91	27
Black women	0.17	6	0.24	8	0.54	23
Age (Years)						
< 50	0.06	36	0.07	44	0.14	98
50–59	0.27	22	0.69	61	0.69	60
60–69	0.81	46	0.89	58	1.21	86
≥ 70	0.92	44	1.15	65	1.66	101
Registration Date						
Whites						
San Francisco	0.32	37	0.27	32	0.45	53
Detroit	0.18	23	0.26	35	0.48	62
Connecticut	0.17	21	0.21	27	0.42	55
Blacks						
San Francisco	0.57	7	0.83	11	0.79	11
Detroit	0.24	7	0.36	10	0.90	28
Connecticut	0.63	3	0.69	4	0.81	7
Total	0.20	148	0.27	228	0.38	345

Note: Data are from the Surveillance, Epidemiology, and End Results Program.

Source: Weinstock, M.A. and Horm, J.W. *JAMA* 60, 42, 1988. With permission.

Only a strong family history of atopic dermatitis in MF patients has been described.[35,36]

Familial cases of CTCL have rarely been reported. Recently, a case of monozygotic twins with CTCL was reported. This study reported that human leukocyte antigens have shown that the histocompatibility antigens HLA-B8, AW3, and AW31 are more frequent in patients with MF.[37]

Analysis of structural chromosome abnormalities in patients with MF reveals that many chromosomes can have clonal abnormalities.[38,39] Chromosome 1 seems to be the most frequently affected: in this the region between 1p22 and 1p36 is thought to contain a gene important in either the malignant transformation or progression of MF.[38]

Also described are different oncogenes, either the NFKB/lyt.10 gene or the tal-1 gene that was mutated in 5 of 38 cases of CTCL.[40] This tal-1 gene codes for a transcription factor that is not expressed in normal T lymphocytes; probably when this is an abnormal deletion of tal-1, it becomes activated and may play a role in malignant transformation.[40]

Some of these results are contradictory. Thus, further research with more cases is needed to clarify the role of familial history in the development of MF.

1.4 RISK FACTORS

1.4.1 OCCUPATIONAL FACTORS

The idea that occupational factors might be involved in the origin of MF fits in quite well with the observation that dermatitis, or more specifically contact dermatitis, may precede the appearance of MF. For example, the operators of different types of machinery are exposed to a wide range of agents such as metals and plastics; they are also exposed to oils used in cutting procedures and to solvents used in grinding operations. Furthermore, some of these agents, which are irritating and sensitizing, have also been recognized as cancer-producing. There are extremely high levels of carcinogenic N-nitrosamine in some makes of fluids used in cutting processes.[32] An appearance of MF has been described following exposure to chemical agents (toxic) caused by industrial accidents.[41]

In a case-control study performed by Cohen et al.,[32] 40 working periods were detected in industry or in the construction industry and were related to 29 of the 59 patients affected by MF (49%). On the other hand, 19 of the 54 controls (35%) were related to industrial jobs, which were comparable to those of the cases (the average duration of the job, both for industrial jobs and for nonindustrial jobs, was similar in the cases and the control subjects).

There were only three instances in which the control subjects had industrial jobs and the cases did not (odds ratio = 4.3; 95% confidence interval). Consequently, the relative risk of finding an industrial occupation among the patients affected by MF was 4.3 times greater than among the control subjects. The association between industrial occupation and MF was statistically significant ($p = .02$).

The main differences between the industrial occupation of the MF patients and the control subjects were found to be among machinists, construction workers, foundry operators, and industrial electricians. These findings indicate that the MF patients were more greatly involved than the heavy industry control subjects. However, some methodological defects were observed in reviewing this study; many of the occupational medical histories were obtained from people close to the patients rather than from the patients themselves, which could account for the biases and errors in classifying the medical histories. The patients affected by MF in this study were employed as machinists, machine operators, textile workers, construction workers, foundry operators, wood industry workers, workers in woodcutting processes, and industrial cleaning service workers (with a greater or lesser frequency). But there were also some in nonindustrial occupations, such as sales staff managers, greater or lesser frequency. Such occupations as mechanics, machinery operators, textile workers, construction workers, and overseers were also found among the control subjects, although less frequently.[32]

Employment in the manufacturing industry, especially petrochemicals, textiles, metals, and machinery, was observed in a descriptive study in 29% of a series of patients ($n = 211$) diagnosed with MF. There were 63 patients (30%) who showed exposure to toxic substances, especially petrochemical substances (11%), metals (7%), and solvents (6%), although there were no data regarding the frequency and the duration of such exposure. No correlation was found between MF and the previous exposure to these toxic substances described.[19]

Between 1961 and 1969 in Sweden, 28 cases were diagnosed among working women (1960 census). The risk significantly increased among women employed in hotel business jobs (hotels and restaurants) (6 cases; SIR = 3.6, adjusted by age and region, $p <.05$), and a high risk was observed in the clothing industry (4 cases; SIR = 2.1).[42]

Additional case-control studies carried out in Scotland, California, and Washington state do not confirm the existence of some type of association between industrial occupation and the risk of MF, but an association was found in Europe (Table 1.6).[43] Recent results from the European study are in line with what other studies have found: that the working activities in the paper and wood industries were carried out in California and Washington. Furthermore, the same studies identify that those cases with a slightly lower socioeconomic level than that of the control subjects are engaged in certain occupations that entail greater exposure to conditions that favor the development of MF, thus supporting the hypothesis that workers of a lower socioeconomic level are at greater risk of developing MF.[31,32]

1.4.2 RADIATION

Exposure to solar radiation defined by episodes of severe sunburn does not reveal any association with MF, although farmworkers, fishing industry workers, and other groups who work out in the open appear to be at greater risk. In a study of 211 patients, 90 burned easily on being exposed to the sun. The data that describe the variations with regard to North–South did not reveal a greater or lesser gradient as far as other skin diseases, such as cutaneous carcinomas and melanomas, are concerned.[19]

One case of MF and several of parapsoriasis were detected among the workers at the Thule Air Base when a military airplane crashed and released plutonium, americium, and tritium in 1968.[44]

No relation has been found between an exposure to x-rays and the appearance of MF.[35] However, more studies and data are needed.

Given the inherent immunological nature of the neoplastic cells responsible for this disorder, it has been proposed that chronic exposure to occupational chemicals, pesticides, or tobacco may predispose individuals to the development of CTCL; however, none of these potential associations has survived scrutiny.[30,45] The observations that the disease is more common in African Americans than in whites and that it often presents firstly in areas normally shielded from the sun (i.e., the "bathing trunk" distribution) collectively suggest that actinic exposure may actually inhibit

TABLE 1.6
Odds Ratios for Mycosis Fungoides in Participants Who Have Always Worked in Industries[a] Represented with at Least Two Exposed Cases

NACE Code	Description	Cases	Controls	OR[b]	95% Confidence Interval
	Male				
26	Manufacture of other nonmetallic mineral products	4	21	5.3	1.7–16.2
51	Wholesale trade and commission trade	3	46	3.6	1.2–10.5
63	Transport activities	2	17	3.4	0.8–15.3
65	Financial intermediation, except insurance and pension funding	3	31	3.0	0.9–10.5
80	Primary school	2	46	2.1	0.5–9.1
75	Public administration	3	102	1.7	0.6–4.7
36	Manufacture of furniture, manufacturing	2	44	1.6	0.4–6.8
29	Manufacture of machinery and equipment	3	85	1.3	0.4–4.2
52	Retail trade, except of motor vehicles and motorcycles	2	160	1.2	0.5–3.0
1	Agriculture, hunting and forestry	8	304	0.9	0.4–1.7
	Female				
21	Manufacture of pulp, paper and paper products	2	33	14.4	2.17–95.1
74	Other managerial activities	2	26	4.1	1.3–12.7
18	Manufacture of wearing apparel; dressing and dyeing of fur	4	43	2.4	0.9–6.5
95	Private households with employed persons	4	112	1.8	0.7–4.4
15	Manufacture of food products and beverages	2	33	1.3	0.3–5.5
1	Agriculture, hunting and forestry	5	76	1.1	0.4–2.9
52	Retail trade, except of motor vehicles and motorcycles	4	134	0.9	0.4–2.3

Note: OR, odds ratio.

[a] Industries classified per the Nomenclature of Activities of the European Community, Revision 1, 1993.

[b] ORs adjusted by age, country, and number of jobs.

Source: From Morales Suárez-Varela, M. et al. *J. Occup. Environ. Med.* (in press), 2004. With permission.

the evolution of the malignant clone from normal "cutaneous T cells." It is noteworthy that the epidermotropic collections of CTCL cells, referred to as Pautrier microabscesses, may represent a congregation of malignant T cells around Langerhams cells (LCs), the dendritic antigen-presenting cells (DC) of the epidermis, and that LCs are fairly sensitive to UV damage. This observation has suggested that the epidermotropic CTCL cells may receive growth signals from their contact with LCs. Therefore, it is possible that UV damage of LCs, more significant in whites this growth signal and inhibit the replication of CTCL cells in UV-exposed skin sites. It is also intriguing that the often profound response of patch/plaque CTCL to UV treatment may reflect this phenomenon as well. The observation that individuals infected with the human T-cell leukemia virus type I (HTLV-I) often develop T-cell leukemias with skin involvement, indistinguishable from those of CTCL, has led some to hypothesize that CTCL may be a consequence of infection with HTLV-I, or with another unknown retrovirus, a possibility that remains the subject of active investigation.

1.4.3 LIFESTYLE: ALCOHOL AND TOBACCO CONSUMPTION

In the European Rare Cancer Study, wine had no protective effect and yet, quite to the contrary, the daily consumption of more than 24 g of alcohol was associated with a high risk of MF. There was a dose-dependent increase in the risk of MF with increased smoking habits, although the observed trend was not statistically significant. A combined exposure to high tobacco and alcohol use yielded a significantly increased risk for MF (Table 1.7).[46]

1.4.4 MARITAL STATUS AND LEVEL OF EDUCATION

In the Greene et al.[19] study of 211 MF patients, 75% were married, 14% were widowed, 7% were single, and 4% were divorced. With regard to the patients' educational level, the average number of school years completed was 12 (60% had graduated high school, including 34% whose education went beyond high school).

1.4.5 CUTANEOUS EVOLUTION

In the same study[19] when medical histories were considered in allergic conditions or cutaneous infections, and a history of cancer in the family, exposures to toxic substances, an occupation in the manufacturing industries, and sensitivity to the sun were all examined as possible risk factors, it was found that 18 of the 211 patients (8%) did not present any risk factor. Among the remaining 92%, 168 (80%) presented with two or more risk factors, and 108 (51%) presented with three or more risk factors.

Generally speaking, if there was any type of allergy demonstrated by cutaneous tests, no differences were found between cases and controls. By means of the medical histories, Cohen et al.'s study[32] was able to verify that many patients affected by MF had histories of rashes prior to diagnosis, mainly nonspecific rashes or dermatitis, and also contact dermatitis, although less frequently, and even mucinosis.[69] Some patients had atopic or nummular eczema, psoriasis, and contact dermatitis including a general exfoliative dermatitis, with a greater or lesser frequency.[47]

Personal histories of contact dermatitis, asthma, rhinitis, or atopic dermatitis have not been related to an increase in the risk of MF; although significant differences were seen in the association between family medical histories of atopic dermatitis and a greater risk of suffering from the disease. A family medical history of benign inflammatory dermatosis appears to be a risk factor for MF,[36] but its study has proven

TABLE 1.7

Odds Ratios[a] for Mycosis Fungoides According to the Combined Use of Wine and Tobacco[b] (with 95% Confidence Intervals in Parentheses)[46]

Wine intake (grams alcohol/day)	Tobacco Use (Pack Years)									Tobacco Use Adjusted for Wine Intake
	0			1–24 (Up to 2 Units per Day)			>24 (More than 2 Units per Day)			
	Cases	Controls	OR	Cases	Controls	OR	Cases	Controls	OR	OR
0	11	348	1.0	26	797	1.93 (0.90–4.10)	1	90	0.42 (0.05–3.47)	1.0
1–25		193	0.41 (0.05–3.33)	14	617	1.71 (0.70–4.14)	3	81	1.75 (0.43–7.08)	0.92 (0.50–1.70)
>25	1	191	0.45 (0.06–3.69)	15	441	2.47 (1.0–6.10)	4	140	1.25 (0.35–4.45)	1.19 (0.64–2.23)
Wine intake adjusted for tobacco use			1.0			2.41 (1.26–4.63)			1.29 (0.49–3.40)	76 cases/ 2899 controls

Note: OR, odds ratio.

[a] Adjusted for country, age, sex, and education. Logistic regression.

[b] The table for definite and possible cases combined.

Source: From Morales Suárez-Varela, M. et al. *Eur. J. Cancer* 37, 392, 2001. With permission.

TABLE 1.8

Odds Ratios for Definitive and Possible Cases of Mycosis Fungoides According to Infection or Atopic Dermatitis Reported Present 5 Years before Mycosis Fungoides Was Diagnosed

	Cases			Definitive Cases			Possible Cases		
	Definitive	Possible	Controls	ORc	ORa	95% CI	ORc	ORa	95% CI
Infection									
No	18	8	733	1	1	Ref.	1	1	Ref.
All	36	14	1367	1.1	1.5	0.8–2.7	1.0	1.3	0.6–3.2
Dermatitis									
No	53	19	2276	1	1	Ref.	1	1	Ref.
Yes	13	7	417	1.4	1.6	0.8–3.0	2.0	2.3	0.9–5.5

Note: All, mumps or herpes or hepatitis; ORc, crude odds ratio; ORa, odds ratio adjusted by sex, age, and country; CI, confidence interval. Missing data on infection or dermatitis were excluded.

Source: From Morales Suárez-Varela, M. *Eur. J. Cancer* 39, 511, 2003. With permission.

1.4.6 OTHER RISK FACTORS

Some MF cases caused by organ transplants or by HIV infection have been described in immunodepressed patients,[48] although this appears to be infrequent.[49]

Occasionally, lesions similar to those produced by CTCL have been observed in AIDS patients.[50] Patients infected with HIV concomitantly with CTCL, even in the absence of a severe immunodepression, develop an atypical course of the disease, and its progress is more rapid.[51]

Although there are different hypotheses regarding the etiology of MF (viral agents or an alteration in the cellular immunity), if other benign diseases with similar clinical characteristics are compared (dermatosis, parapsoriasis, eczema, etc.), the main hypothesis continues to be that of the alteration in cellular immunity.

In the European multicenter case-control study, information on infections, skin pathology, and clinical history 5 years before the diagnosis of MF was used to estimate the risk of MF. The highest risk was found in patients who reported a history of psoriasis 5 years before the diagnosis. Infections and atopic diseases were not closely associated. Whether this can be a causal background or simply reflects early diagnostic uncertainty is not known (Table 1.8).[52]

In a study carried out by Fischmann et al.,[53] among 43 patients affected by MF or by Sezary syndrome, 86% were regular smokers, 20% habitually used painkillers, 18% used tranquilizers, and 14% used thiazides.

There appears to be no evidence that marital status, mobility (taking journeys), the use of drugs, exposure to UV light, alcohol consumption, or smoking habits are related to MF.[34–36] Nevertheless, according to the Fischmann et al. study,[53] those patients with chronic cutaneous pathologies, and who have been exposed to a combination of chemical, physical, and biological agents for a long time, who smoke a lot and who have

1.5 MORTALITY AND SURVIVAL

In the United States fewer than 100 deaths a year[46] are attributed on average to this neoplasm. In the period between 1950 and 1975 (excluding 1972), 1948 deaths were attributed to MF (Table 1.6). The annual average rates of mortality, specified by age, revealed a greater rate in men than in women, and a similar difference was found between nonwhites and whites. The annual average rate of mortality, adjusted by age, according to race, during this 25-year period, was as follows: white men, 0.53 × 10⁶; white women, 0.28 × 10⁶; nonwhite men, 0.84 × 10⁶; and nonwhite women, 0.54 × 10⁶. The mortality rate increases with age, with a mortality peak found between 65 and 69 years of age for men from the nonwhite race and between 75 and 84 years of age for men from the white race.[19]

In data for the United States between 1950 and 1975, greater mortality rates were observed among white men and in urban areas in the Northeast. No consistent difference was noted with respect to socioeconomic level. Mortality was greater in the counties that had the following industries: oil, rubber, metal, machinery, and printing,[19] although no consistent difference was noted as far as socioeconomic level is concerned.

In summary, the survival of patients with MF and other forms of CTCL depends on accurate diagnosis and effective treatment, but these areas continue to present a challenge for clinicians. There are a multitude of clinical and histopathological presentations of MF (more than 20 forms have been described) as well as a variety of therapeutic options, with a lack of randomized trials to establish efficacy with adequate epidemiological surveillance.

ACKNOWLEDGMENTS

I am indebted to Dr. M.A. Weinstock for help in the preparation of the manuscript and to Dr. H. Zackheim for his generous assistance and helpful comments. Thanks also to Prof. J. Olsen from Aarhus University and Dr. S. Ferrer from Valencia.

REFERENCES

1. Zackheim, H.S. and McCalmont, T.H. Mycosis fungoides: the great imitator. *J. Am. Dermatol.* 47, 914, 2002.
2. Alibert, J.L.M. *Description des Maladies de la Peau Observées à l'Hôpital St. Louis.* Barrois L'aire et Fils, Paris, 1806, p. 413.
3. Bazin, P.A.E. *Maladies de la Peau Observées à l'Hôpital St. Louis.* Paris, 1876.
4. Lutzner, M.A. et al. Cutaneous T-cell lymphomas: The Sezary syndrome, MF and related disorders. *Ann. Intern. Med.* 83, 534, 1975.
5. Berger, C.L. et al. Dual genotype in cutaneous T cell lymphoma: immunoglobulin gene rearrangement in clonal T cell. *J. Invest. Dermatol.* 90, 73, 1988.
6. Harris, N.L. et al. A revised European–American classification of lymphoid neoplasms: a proposal from the International Lymphoma Study Group. *Blood,* 84, 1361, 1994.
7. Willenze, R. et al. EORTC classification for primary cutaneous lymphomas: a proposal from the Cutaneous Lymphoma Study Group of the European Organization for

8. The Non-Hodgkin's Lymphoma Pathologic Classification Project. National Cancer Institute-sponsored study of classifications of non-Hodgkin's lymphomas: summary and description of working formulation for clinical usage. *Cancer*, 49, 2112, 1982.

9. Weinstock, M.A. and Horm, J.W. Mycosis fungoides in the United States. *JAMA* 60, 42, 1988.

10. Wilson, L.D. Personal communication regarding the Surveillance, Epidemiology, and End Results (SEER) Program, National Cancer Institute. 1995.

11. Hartmann, T.B. et al. Serex identification of new tumour associated antigens in cutaneous T-cell lymphoma. *Br. J. Dermatol.* 150, 252, 2004.

12. Storm, H.H. et al. Cancer incidence in Denmark 1987. Copenhagen: Danish Cancer Society. *Danish Cancer Registry*, 1990.

13. McFadden, N. et al. Mycosis fungoides in Norway 1960–1980. *Act. Dermato. Veneorol.* 109, 1, 1983.

14. Burns, M.K., Ellis, C.N., and Cooper, K.D. Mycosis fungoide-type cutaneous T-cell lymphoma arising before 30 years of age: inmunophenotypic, inmunogenotypic and clinicopathologic analysis of nine cases. *J. Am. Acad. Dermatol.* 6, 974, 1992.

15. Koch, S.E. et al. Mycosis fungoides beginning in childhood and adolescence. *J. Am. Acad. Dermatol.* 17, 563, 1987.

16. Peters, M.S. et al. Mycosis fungoides in children and adolescents. *J. Am. Acad. Dermatol.* 22, 1011, 1990.

17. Wilson, A.G.M. et al. Mycosis fungoides in childhood: An unusual presentation. *J. Am. Acad. Dermatol.* 25, 370, 1991.

18. Zackheim, H.S. et al. Mycosis fungoides with onset before 20 years of age. *J. Am. Acad. Dermatol.* 36, 557, 1997.

19. Greene, M.H. et al. Mycosis fungoides: Epidemiologic observations. *Cancer Treat. Rep.* 63, 597, 1979.

20. Orkin, M., Maibach, H.I., and Dahl, M.V. *Dermatologia* Ed. El Manual Moderno. Méjico 651, 7, 1994.

21. Bernstein, L., Deapen, D., and Ross, R.K. Mycosis fungoides. *JAMA* 261, 1882, 1989.

22. Yang, K. et al. T-cell lymphoma. *Nat. Can. Inst. Monogr.* 69, 35, 1989.

23. Weinstock, M.A. and Gadstein, B. Twenty year trends in the reported incidence and mortality of mycosis fungoides. *Am. J. Public Health* 89, 1240, 1999.

24. Kim, Y.H. et al. Prognostic factors in erythrodermic mycosis fungoides and the Sezary syndrome. *Arch. Dermatol.* 131, 1003, 1995.

25. Weiss, L.M. et al. Clonal rearrangements of T-cell receptor genes in mycosis fungoides and dermatopathic lymphadenopathy. *New England J. Med.* 313, 539, 1985.

26. Rook, A.H. and Heald, P. The immunopathogenesis of cutaneous T-cell lymphoma. *Hematol./Oncol. Clin. North Am.* 9, 997, 1995.

27. Dalloul, A. et al. Interleukin-7 is a growth factor for Sézary lymphoma cells. *J. Clin. Invest.* 90, 1054, 1992.

28. Rich, B.E. et al. Cutaneous lymphoproliferation and lymphomas on interleukin 7 transgenic mice. *J. Exp. Med.* 177, 305, 1993.

29. Rowden, G. and Lewis, M.G. Langerhans cells: Involvement in the pathogenesis of mycosis fungoides. *Br. J. Dermatol.* 95, 665, 1976.

30. Tan, R.A. et al. Mycosis fungoides, a disease of antigen persistence. *Br. J. Dermatol.* 91, 607, 1974.

31. Weinstock, M.A. Epidemiology of mycosis fungoide. *Seminars in Dermatol.* 13(3), 154, 1994.

32. Cohen, S.R. et al. Clinicopathologic relationships, survival, and therapy in 59 patients

33. Berkson, J. Limitations of the application of fourfold table analysis to hospital data. *Biometrics,* 2, 47, 1946.
34. Weinstock, M.A. A registred-based case-control study of mycosis fungoide. *Ann. Epidemiol.* 1(5), 533, 1991.
35. Whittemore, A.S. and Holly, E.A. Mycosis fungoide in relation to environmental exposures and inmune response: a case-control study. *J. Natl. Cancer. Inst.* 18, 81(20), 1560, 1989.
36. Tuyp, E. et al. A case-control study of possible causative factors in mycosis fungoides. *Arch. Dermatol.* 123, 196, 1987.
37. Schneider, B.F. et al. Familial occurrence of cutaneous T-cell lymphoma: A case report of monozygotic twin sisters. *Leukemia,* 9, 1979, 1995.
38. Thangavelu, M. et al. Recurring structural chromosome abnormalities in peripheral blood lymphocytes of patients with mycosis fungoides/Sézary syndrome. *Blood,* 89, 3371, 1997.
39. Limon, J. et al. Chromosome aberrations, spontaneous SCE, and growth kinetics in PHA-stimulated lymphocytes of five cases with Sézary syndrome. *Cancer Genet. Cytogenet.* 83, 75, 1995.
40. Neri, A. et al. Molecular analysis of cutaneous B and T-cell lymphomas. *Blood,* 86, 3160, 1995.
41. Lambert, W.C., Cohen, P.J., and Schwartz, R.A. Surgical management of mycosis fungoides. *J. Med.* 28(3–4), 211, 1997.
42. Linet, M.S. et al. Occupation and hematopoietic and lymphoproliferative malignancies among women: a linked registry study. *J. Occup. Med.* 36, 1187, 1994.
43. Morales Suárez-Varela, M. et al. Occupational risk factors for mycosis fungoides: A European multicenter case-control study. *J. Occup. Environ. Med.* (in press), 2004.
44. Zachariae, H. and Sogaard, H. Plutonium-induced mycosis fungoides and parapsoriasis en plaques — a new entity? *Curr. Probl. Dermatol.* 19, 81, 1990.
45. Olivan Ballabriga, A., Reparaz Prados, J., and Sala Boneta, J. Micosis fungoide asociada a infecció por VIH. *Anales de Medicina Interna* 7(2), 83, 1990.
46. Morales Suárez-Varela, M. et al. Are alcohol intake and smoking associated with mycosis fungoides? A European multicentre case-control study. *Eur. J. Cancer* 37, 392, 2001.
47. King, I.D. and Ackerman, A.B. Guttate Parapsoriasis/Digitate dermatosis (small plaque parapsoriasis) is mycosis fungoides. *Am. J. Dermatol.* 14, 518, 1992.
48. Nahass, G.T. and Kraffert, C.A. Cutaneous T-cell lymphoma associated with the acquired immunodeficiency syndrome. *Arch. Dermatol.* 127, 1020, 1991.
49. Sorrells, T. et al. Spontaneous regression of granulomatous mycosis fungoides in an HIV positive patient. *J. Am. Acad. Dermatol.* 37, 876, 1997.
50. Lorincz, A.L. Cutaneous T-cell lymphoma (mycosis fungoides). *Lancet* 347, 871, 1996.
51. Burns, M.K. and Cooper, K.D. Cutaneus T-cell lymphoma associated with HIV infection. *J. Am. Acad. Dermatol.* 29, 394, 1993.
52. Morales Suárez-Varela, M. Viral infection, atopy and mycosis fungoides: A European multicentre case-control study. *Eur. J. Cancer* 39, 511, 2003.
53. Fischmann, A.B. et al. Exposure to chemicals, physical agents, and biologic agents in mycosis fungoides and the Sezary syndrome. *Cancer Treat. Rep.* 63, 591, 1979.

2 Mycosis Fungoides: Clinical Features

Herschel S. Zackheim

CONTENTS

2.1 MYCOSIS FUNGOIDES PATCH STAGE

The earliest stage of mycosis fungoides (MF) is the patch stage. Patch-stage lesions are typically thin, noninfiltrated, pink, and slightly scaly (Figures 2.1–2.3). Most lesions range from about 2 to 6 cm, but they may be smaller or much larger. The sites of predilection are the sun-protected areas such as the buttocks, hips, lower abdomen, groins, breasts, and inner extremities. Conversely, patch-stage lesions are relatively uncommon on sun-exposed areas such as the face and dorsa of the hands. Nevertheless, lesions may appear on any part of the body surface. Patch-stage lesions may be atrophic. When atrophic lesions exhibit telangiectasia and pigmentation, the term "poikiloderma" is used (Figures 2.4 and 2.5).

Another type of patch-stage MF that has been recognized more in recent years is the hypopigmented form.[1] This affects primarily dark-skinned patients. The lesions may present as macules, patches, or thin plaques (Figure 2.6). Hypopigmented MF is relatively more common in young persons as compared to ordinary patch-stage MF. Lesions are predominantly on the trunk, in contrast to vitiligo, which is more often on the extremities and face. Hypopigmented MF lesions, particularly in young persons, also are generally smaller size than in vitiligo and are more apt to be confused with tinea versicolor.

Overall, patch-stage lesions are asymptomatic or mildly pruritic. However, they may be markedly pruritic in some patients.

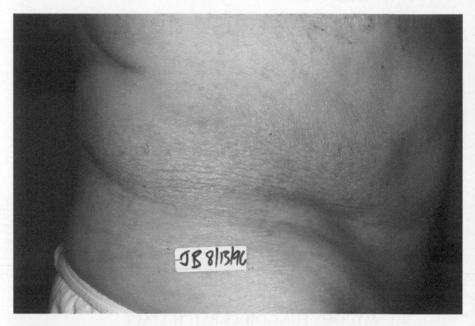

FIGURE 2.1 (See color insert following page 18.) Patch-stage mycosis fungoides on the lower flank.

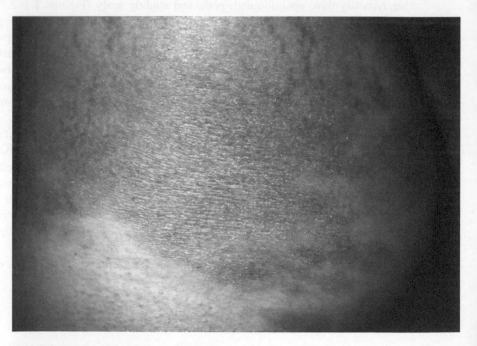

FIGURE 2.2 (See color insert.) Patch-stage mycosis fungoides on the lateral buttocks.

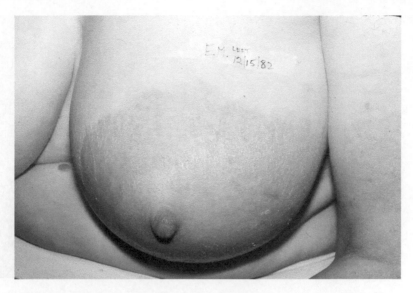

FIGURE 2.3 Patch-stage mycosis fungoides on the breast.

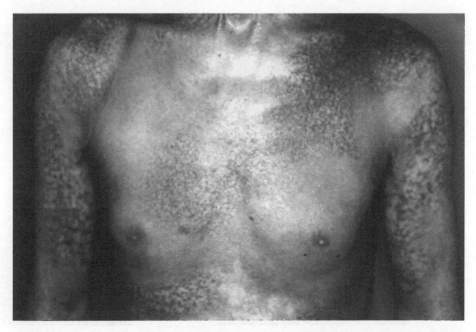

FIGURE 2.4 (See color insert.) Almost universal poikilodermatous mycosis fungoides. There is atrophy, telangiectasia, and pigmentation.

FIGURE 2.5 Close view of poikiloderma.

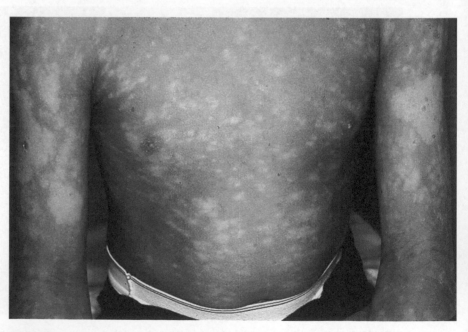

FIGURE 2.6 **(See color insert.)** Extensive hypopigmented mycosis fungoides.

2.2 MF PLAQUE STAGE

Plaque-stage lesions are generally flat, indurated, and elevated above the skin surface (Figures 2.7–2.9). Lesions are usually 2 to 5 cm in diameter, but they may be larger or may present as small papules. Any area of the body surface may be involved. Plaque-stage lesions are mostly asymptomatic or mildly pruritic, although pruritus may be severe.

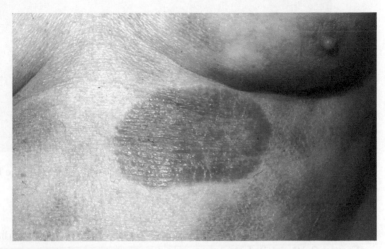

FIGURE 2.7 Sharply defined plaque-stage lesion of mycosis fungoides.

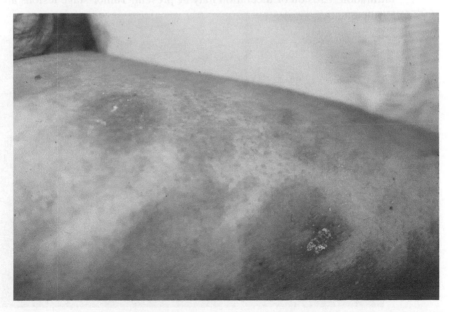

FIGURE 2.8 (See color insert.) Multiple lesions of plaque-stage mycosis fungoides on the thigh.

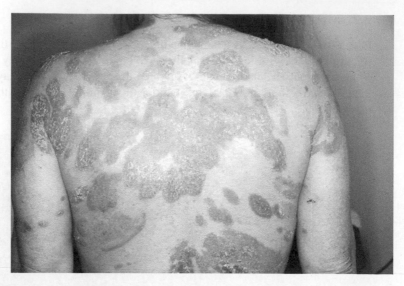

FIGURE 2.9 Extensive lesions of plaque-stage mycosis fungoides on the back.

2.3 MF TUMOR STAGE

Tumor-stage MF most commonly presents as nodules 1 to 3 cm in diameter or larger (Figures 2.10–2.12). Less commonly, tumor stage presents as a poorly defined deep infiltration. Erosion or ulceration may be present. Tumor-stage lesions are relatively asymptomatic.

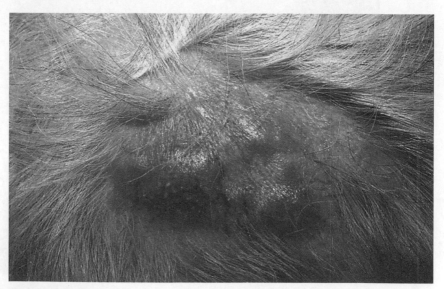

FIGURE 2.10 (See color insert.) Nodules of tumor-stage mycosis fungoides on the scalp.

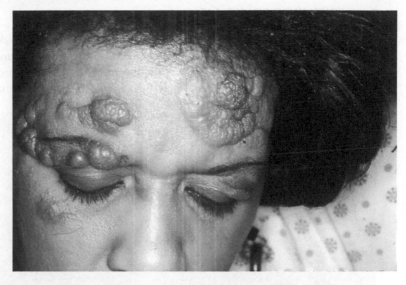

FIGURE 2.11 Nodules and infiltrated plaques of tumor-stage mycosis fungoides on the face.

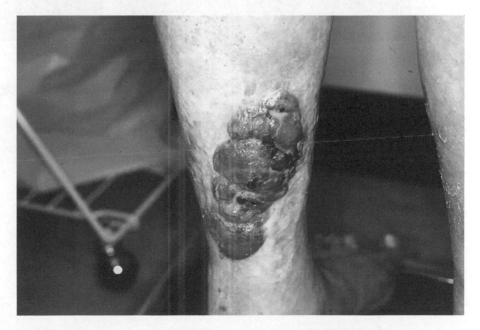

FIGURE 2.12 (See color insert.) Exuberant mycosis fungoides tumor on the leg.

2.4 ERYTHRODERMIC MF

Erythrodermic MF presents as widespread erythema. The involved skin is pink or bright red. Most often the erythematous skin is diffusely scaly (Figure 2.13), but it may be purely macular. Characteristically, the palms and soles are erythematous, usually scaly or hyperkeratotic, and may be painfully fissured (Figure 2.14).

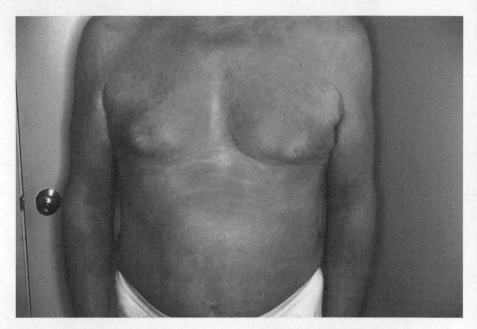

FIGURE 2.13 (See color insert.) Universal erythroderma.

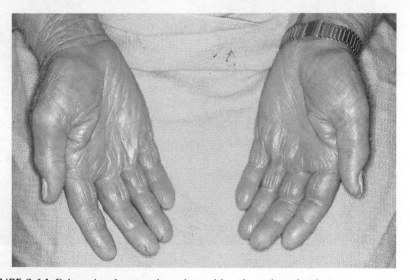

FIGURE 2.14 Palmar involvement in patient with universal erythroderma.

Generalized pruritus is usually the most distressing symptom in erythrodermic MF. This pruritus may be very intense and is usually difficult to control. The patient commonly feels chilly as a result of loss of heat through the impaired barrier of the exfoliative skin. Another troublesome symptom is painful, fissured palms.

Differentiation from Sezary syndrome depends on whether or not there is evidence of blood involvement (see Chapter 4, "Sezary Syndrome").

REFERENCES

1. Akaraphanth, R., Douglass, M.C., and Lim, H.W. Hypopigmented mycosis fungoides: treatment and a 6-year follow-up of 9 patients. *J. Am. Acad. Dermatol.* 42, 33, 2000.

3 Mycosis Fungoides: Histopathology

Anne E. Wilkerson and Bruce R. Smoller

CONTENTS

3.1 INTRODUCTION

Cutaneous T-cell lymphomas (CTCLs) are a heterogenous group of T-cell neoplasms that display a variety of clinical and histopathological presentations. Included in the Revised European-American Lymphoma/World Health Organization classification of primary CTCLs are mycosis fungoides (MF) and MF variants, pagetoid reticulosis, large cell CTCL, which includes the more indolent CD30+ anaplastic large cell lymphoma (ALCL) and the more aggressive CD30– variant, lymphomatoid papulosis, and subcutaneous panniculitis-like T-cell lymphoma. Each of these demonstrates a range of clinical and histologic features, genetic abnormalities, prognoses, and responses to treatment. MF is the most common form of T-cell lymphoma, and the term is often used interchangeably with T-cell lymphoma. However, MF is a unique form of T-cell lymphoma that describes a disease that typically progresses clinically through patch, plaque, and tumor stages and possibly erythroderma. The histology varies according to these stages, with diagnosis of the early lesions remaining a major challenge for pathologists without T-cell clonality studies due to the slow evolution of the disease.[1] Efforts have been made to establish consistent diagnostic criteria for MF to allow for more definitive diagnoses. These have included evaluating the density of the lymphocytic infiltrate, presence and extent of epidermotropism of lymphocytes, and degree of lymphocytic atypia.[1] Of these features, nuclear atypia of the lymphocytes was the feature least consistently agreed upon by pathologists; however, applying consistent diagnostic criteria nearly doubled the likelihood of a definitive diagnosis of MF.[1] In this chapter, these histologic features of classical MF in the various clinical stages, as well as the major histologic variants, are discussed.

3.2 HISTOPATHOLOGY

MF is divided into patch, plaque, and tumor stages depending on the clinical presentation of the patient. Patients presenting early in the disease are often in the patch stage and may subsequently progress to the plaque and tumor stages. This occurs in a minority of cases. Although some cases may not be definitely placed in one of these three clinical stages solely on histologic criteria, the histologic findings often correlate well with the clinical stage of the patient. Diagnosis of the earliest stages of disease relies more on the architectural features of the infiltrate, with the later stages of the disease demonstrating more cytologic atypia of the lymphocytes. Therefore, recognition of the earliest presentations requires a higher index of clinical and histologic suspicion. Furthermore, one must recognize possible alterations of the histology of MF due to various treatment modalities.

3.2.1 PATCH STAGE

As mentioned above, patients presenting at the earliest stage of MF, often with only slightly scaly, erythematous patches, may prove diagnostically challenging.[1-11] As the histologic features of early patch-stage MF are subtle and may appear as one of many superficial inflammatory lesions, early biopsies may not be definitely diagnosed as MF. Multiple attempts have been made to establish consistent, minimal histologic criteria for the early diagnosis of MF; however, a consensus of minimal criteria has not been reached, partly due to the overlap and variety of histology of the different stages of MF.[1-5,7,9,10,12,13]

The classical histologic findings in the patch stage of MF include a variably dense, bandlike dermal infiltrate of small to medium lymphocytes along the basal layer of the epidermis with migration of these cells into the epidermis (epidermotropism; Figure 3.1a and 3.1b). Lymphocytes involving the epidermis are present as single cells and/or small collections of cells lining the basal layer of the epidermis with few scattered lymphocytes within the epidermis.[14] These intraepidermal lymphocytes are often larger and more atypical than the lymphocytes lining the basilar layer. Epidermotropic lymphocytes higher in the epidermis may also be distinguished by having a prominent clear halo that surrounds the nuclei of the

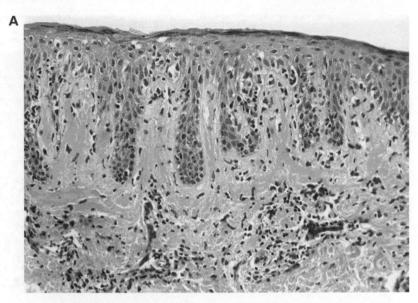

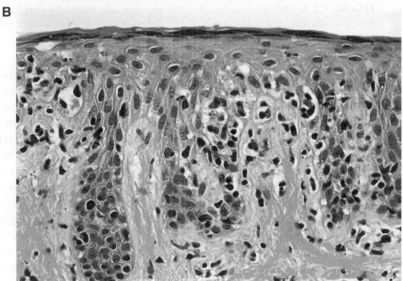

FIGURE 3.1 (a) Low-power view (H&E, 10×) of patch-stage mycosis fungoides (MF), demonstrating an epidermis with mild psoriasiform hyperplasia and epidertropism of medium sized lymphocytes. (b) Higher power view (H&E, 20×) of patch-stage MF, illustrating lymphocytes lining the dermo-epidermal junction in early patch-stage MF. Also note small collections of two to three lymphocytes within epidermis, some of which are surrounded by clear halos.

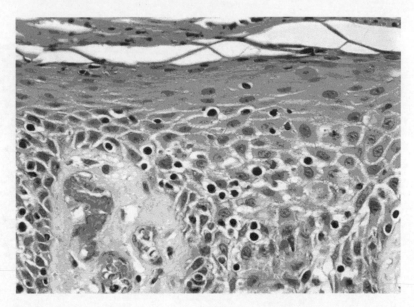

FIGURE 3.2 Epidermotropic lymphocytes are often surrounded by clear halos in patch-stage mycosis fungoides (MF) and are useful in distinguishing MF from other inflammatory dermatoses (H&E, 20×).

lymphocytes, thus separating the cell from the surrounding keratinocytes (Figure 3.2). This feature may prove one of the most helpful distinguishing features of infiltrates in MF compared to non-MF cases.[15] Typically, the epidermis is only mildly spongiotic, especially when considering the amount of epidermotropism, and may demonstrate mild psoriasiform hyperplasia or atrophy. Dyskeratotic cells are not typical of the patch stage of MF. Although Pautrier's microabscesses, defined as discreet collections of atypical lymphocytes within the epidermis, are considered very sensitive for all stages of MF, they are actually more common in the plaque stage, being present in less than 10% of cases in the patch stage of the disease (Figure 3.3). The dermal infiltrate may involve both the papillary dermis and superficial reticular dermis; however, unlike the plaque and tumor stages, mitotic figures are rare. The papillary dermis is often nonspecifically fibrotic and contains a variably dense lymphocytic infiltrate, which may be either minimal or more moderate in a perivascular or bandlike distribution.[8,16] The infiltrate may include rare eosinophils and plasma cells, and pigment incontinence can be seen. Immunohistochemistry demonstrates that the neoplastic lymphocytes are CD2+, CD3+, CD4+, CD45RO+, and CD8−.[17,18] The majority of the cells are CD30− and often also CD7−. Some authors include lesions with CD8+ epidermotropic lymphocytes as MF (cytotoxic immunophenotype variant).[19] However, as these lesions tend to behave more aggressively and offer a worse prognosis, these cases are best not classified as MF and should be separated as CD8+ epidermotropic T-cell lymphoma.[19] Additionally, scattered B cells may be occasionally present in the infiltrate in MF.

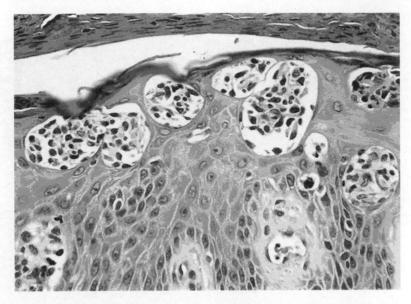

FIGURE 3.3 Pautrier's microabscess consists of collections of medium to large lymphocytes within the epidermis, as demonstrated in this case of plaque-stage mycosis fungoides (H&E, 20×). Also note occasional single epidermotropic lymphocytes with clear halos within this psoriasiform epidermis.

3.2.2 PLAQUE STAGE

As patients progress from the patch to plaque stages, they develop a heavier infiltrate of atypical lymphocytes with the more classic histologic findings of MF.[10,20] Therefore, these more intense lesions are typically easier to diagnosis than those in the patch stage.[6,8,12,13,18] In this stage, there are numerous larger epidermotropic lymphocytes with prominent clear halos forming a dense bandlike infiltrate along the basal layer of the epidermis (Figure 3.4). Pautrier's microabscesses are more likely to be identified in the plaque stage than the patch stage; however, these may be present in only half of the biopsies. The epidermis may demonstrate focal parakeratosis, mild spongiosis, atrophy, or psoriasiform hyperplasia.[5,21] Lymphocytes usually display more nuclear atypia than seen in the patch stage of the disease, with the nuclei appearing more hyperchromatic, cerebriform or indented. Mitotic figures may be seen within dermis. Additionally, plaque-stage lesions show more papillary dermal fibrosis than seen in the newer patch-stage lesions, and the infiltrate may extend into the deeper reticular dermis. Plasma cells and eosinophils are also more common in this stage of the disease.

3.2.3 TUMOR STAGE

The tumor stage of MF is characterized by a dense infiltrate of large lymphocytes filling the dermis and lacking the cytologic and architectural features of the patch and plaque stages of the disease. Architectural distinctions from the earlier stages of

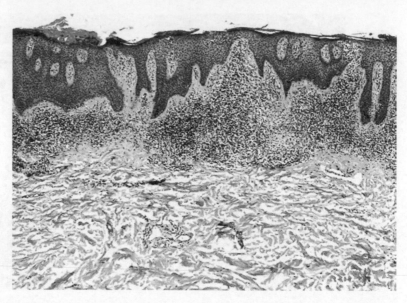

FIGURE 3.4 Patch-stage mycosis fungoides (H&E, 4×) demonstrates a bandlike infiltrate of medium sized lymphocytes with overlying psoriasiform hyperplasia.

MF include neoplastic lymphocytes filling the dermis, extending deeper than in the patch or plaque stage to form nodules in the deep dermis or subcutis, and the lack of epidermal or appendeal infiltration by these neoplastic cells (Figure 3.5). Cytologically, these lymphocytes lack the cerebriform and indented nuclei of the earlier stages and appear more monomorphic, larger, vesiculated nuclei and prominent, often multiple nucleoli.[6,8,12,13,18,22] As expected, mitotic figures are common and may be atypical. Compared to the patch stage, tumor cells are also more likely to be CD7– and CD30+ in the tumor stage of MF. In summary, the cytologic and architectural features of the neoplastic lymphocytes may make accurate distinction from other forms of cutaneous lymphoma very difficult without proper clinical history.

The *d'emblée* form of MF is a term historically referring to cases in which the tumor stage appeared to arise de novo. However, studies have demonstrated that the large neoplastic infiltrates in these lesions are mostly CD30+ lymphocytes.[23,24] Therefore, these cases are currently best classified as primary cutaneous large cell anaplastic lymphoma rather than MF.

3.3 OTHER VARIANTS OF MF

3.3.1 Folliculotropic (Folliculocentric, Adnexotropic, Pilotropic) Variant

The folliculotropic variant of MF is a recently recognized form of MF characterized by mildly epidermotropic neoplastic lymphocytes with pronounced infiltration of the follicular and/or eccrine structures (Figure 3.6).[25–34] Sebaceous glands may be

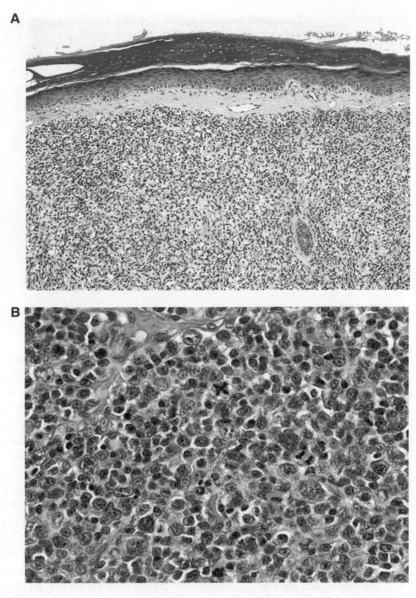

FIGURE 3.5 (a) Tumor-stage mycosis fungoides (MF; H&E, 10×) lacks several of the characteristics of patch and plaque-stage MF, demonstrating minimal epidermal changes including epidermotropic lymphocytes and Pautrier's microabscesses. There is a grenz zone separating the neoplastic lymphocytes in the dermis from the overlying spared epidermis. The dermal infiltrate is composed of atypical lymphocytes admixed with occasional histiocytes. (b) A higher power view of the predominantly dermal infiltrate of atypical lymphocytes in the tumor stage of MF (H&E, 40×). Note pleomorphism of the large neoplastic cells with atypical nuclear contours and several mitotic figures, one of which is atypical.

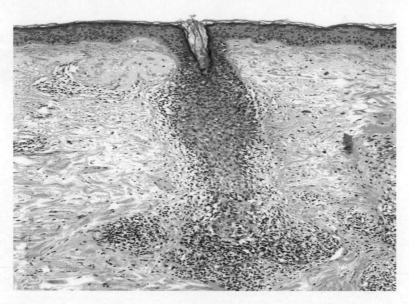

FIGURE 3.6 This low-power view of folliculocentric mycosis fungoides (H&E, 4×) shows a relatively spared epidermis and a brisk perifollicular infiltrate within the dermis.

may appear dilated with keratin plugs and form infundibular cysts.[25,26] The lymphocytes usually display the same cytologic atypia characteristic of the usual subtypes of MF; however, there may only be minor atypia, making gene rearrangements especially helpful in such cases.[27] This test may be necessary to exclude lupus erythematosus or lichen planopilaris in some cases. The follicular epithelium may be minimally spongiotic and contain a dense infiltrate of neoplastic lymphocytes, some of which may form collections similar to Pautrier's microabscesses. Eosinophils may also be present in the infiltrate as well as mucin deposition. Deposition of mucin may make distinction from follicular mucinosis-like MF unclear, therefore, it has been suggested this subtype should be grouped together with follicular mucinosis-like MF.[28] Currently, however, these cases are considered as a separate clinical entity. As folliculotropic MF may be more difficult to treat clinically, recognizing this variant may be helpful prognostically. It is postulated that this subtype may be more challenging therapeutically because the neoplastic cells are located deeper in the dermis and are less accessible to treatment than the more typical epidermotropic variants of MF.

3.3.2 Follicular Mucinosis-Like MF

Another subtype of MF is associated with follicular mucinosis. Follicular mucinosis may be idiopathic, which is typically seen in a younger population, or associated with MF in an older population.[35] Similar to and possibly related to the folliculotropic variant, the neoplastic lymphocytic infiltrate of the follicular mucinosis-like variant of MF involves the follicular structures of the dermis with sparing of the epidermis.[36–39] Distinction of this variant from the folliculotropic subtype currently remains with the presence of increased mucin between the keratinocytes of the follicular epithelium (Figure 3.7). The mucin is identified initially at the level of sebaceous glands but may become more diffuse with progressive degeneration. Follicular mucinosis frequently results in destruction of follicular structures and alopecia. An occasional finding in this variant is numerous eosinophils within the follicular epithelium. The cytological features of the typical forms of MF are not always present in these cases. Patients with follicular mucinosis associated MF may have more lesions on the body than those with follicular mucinosis unassociated with lymphoma; however, other criteria to distinguish the cases of MF from idiopathic follicular mucinosis have recently been reported to be ineffective.[35] Therefore, the diagnosis of follicular mucinosis should raise the suspicion of an underlying MF and result in additional studies such as gene rearrangements.[35] As with folliculotropic MF, the deeper nature of the infiltrate may make this variant less responsive to treatment.

3.3.3 HYPOPIGMENTED MF

This variant of MF presents clinically with hypopigmented patches in a younger patients with darker complexions.[40] Histologically, these lesions are essentially indistinguishable from normal patch-stage lesions that appear clinically as erythematous or hyper pigmented patches.[40] Biopsy of the hypopigmented patches reveals an epidermotropic infiltrate of atypical lymphocytes with the added histologic finding of prominent pigment incontinence.[40–42] In many ways, the neoplastic infiltrate is relatively scant, making the diagnosis difficult. These may contain more CD8+ lymphocytes than typical cases of MF.

3.3.4 GRANULOMATOUS MF

Granulomatous MF is an unusual variant distinguished by the presence of granulomatous foci within an atypical infiltrate of lymphocytes within the papillary dermis and superficial reticular dermis.[44–47] The histiocytes may be arranged in a palisading and interstitial pattern with interstitial lymphocytes. The neoplastic lymphocytes show the usual atypia of early stages of MF but with variable epidermotropism, which may be a distinguishing feature from granuloma annulare. These granulomas may be tuberculoid in type but lacking caseation,[46] more vaguely formed suggestive of granulomatous slack skin, granuloma annulare, and even leprosy.[44,46,47] The infiltrate may contain huge multinucleated giant cells with innumerous nuclei and possibly containing neoplastic lymphocytes (Figure 3.8).[44] This variant of MF is unusual and may in fact be related to granulomatous slack skin, possibly differentiated by its unusual clinical presentation in the flexoral regions and, histologically, by the deeper granulomatous infiltrate with dermal elastolysis in granulomatous slack skin.[44] Although this variant appears strikingly different than other forms of MF, it is associated with no significant difference in prognosis. As discussed below, granulomatous MF may be related to the interstitial variant of MF.[48]

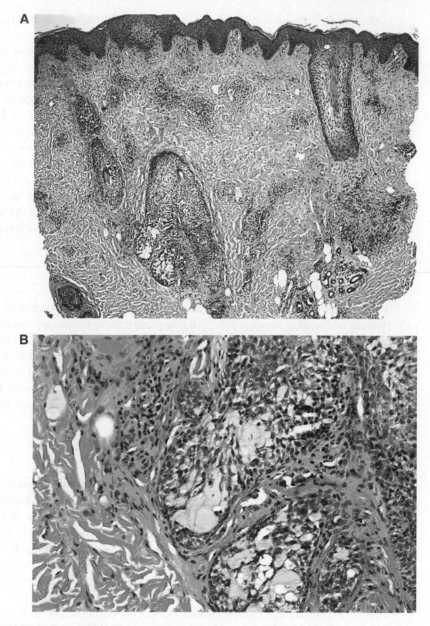

FIGURE 3.7 (a) This low-power view illustrates several follicles within the dermis with focal perifollicular lymphocytes and mucin within the follicle (H&E, 4×). A focally dense interstitial infiltrate of lymphocytes is present in the reticular dermis. The epidermis is predominantly spared. (b) A higher power view highlighting increased mucin within the follicle (H&E, 20×). The adjacent perifollicular infiltrate contains atypical lymphocytes with admixed occasional histiocytes and eosinophils.

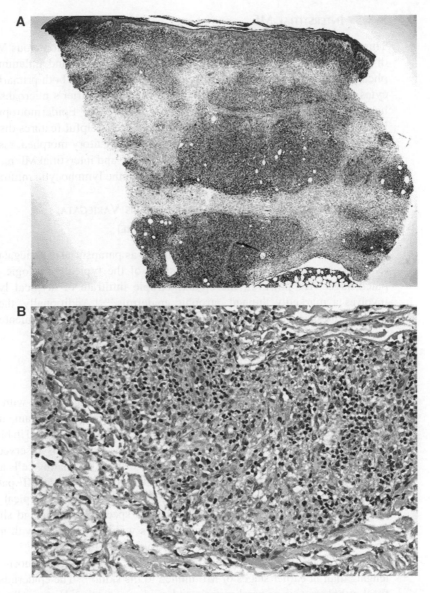

FIGURE 3.8 (a) Granulomatous mycosis fungoides (MF; H&E, 2×) demonstrates palisading histiocytes with admixed atypical lymphocytes extending from the reticular dermis into the deep dermis and subcutis. A brisk bandlike granulomatous infiltrate also involves the papillary dermis with focal mild epidermotropism. (b) A higher power view of granulomatous MF (H&E, 20×) reveals numerous histiocytes with interspersed atypical lymphocytes, resembling other granulomatous processes such as leprosy.

3.3.5 INTERSTITIAL MF

This rarely described variant of MF may be related to granulomatous MF and also displays features of both interstitial granuloma annulare and inflammatory morphea.[49] Histologic sections reveal an interstitial infiltrate of both primarily lymphocytes with scattered histiocytes within the dermis.[49] Pautrier's microabscesses may be observed as well as other histologic features of MF.[49] Epidermotropism and the lack of plasma cells in the dermal infiltrate are both helpful features distinguishing interstitial MF from granuloma annulare and inflammatory morphea, respectively.[49] It has been postulated that both granulomatous MF and interstitial MF may represent a continuum of the host immunologic response to the lymphocytic infiltrate of MF.[49]

3.3.6 POIKILODERMATOUS MF (PARAPSORIASIS VARIEGATA, POIKILODERMA ATROPHICANS VASCULARE)

This variant of MF was previously referred to as parapsoriasis variegata. Histologically, poikilodermatous MF displays some of the typical histologic features of patch-stage MF; however, the epidermotropic infiltrate of atypical lymphocytes involves a markedly thinned, atrophic epidermis.[50,51] Additionally, there may be more pigmentary incontinence similar to that seen in hypopigmented MF and vascular ectasia.[50,51]

3.4 SEZARY SYNDROME

Sezary syndrome is considered to be the leukemic phase of MF, with circulating neoplastic cells that are typically the same size and displaying the same morphology as the neoplastic lymphocytes in MF.[52,53] Sezary cells are highlighted in blood smears by Giemsa and Wright stains. The term Sezary syndrome is reserved for those erythrodermic patients in whom more than 5% of total circulating cells are neoplastic, compared to the less than 5% seen in other erythrodermic MF patients.[52,54,55] Cutaneous findings in Sezary syndrome may rarely include the typical changes of patch or plaque-stage MF; biopsies often lack specific findings and show a more perivascular infiltrate of atypical lymphocytes within the dermis with mild dermal fibrosis and occasional plasma cells and eosinophils (Figure 3.9).[52–56]

Epidermotropism is often minimal or absent, making the diagnosis more challenging than in earlier stages of MF limited to the skin.[52,53] The epidermis may show focal orthokeratosis or parakeratosis and mild spongiosis.[52] Historically, the clinical pattern includes the circulating tumor cells, erythroderma, and lymphadenopathy.[51,54,55]

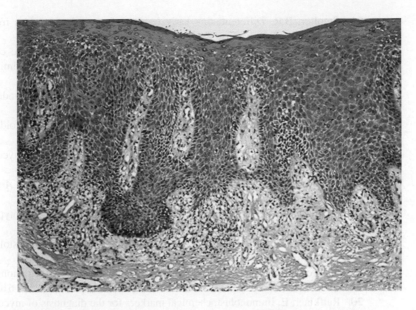

FIGURE 3.9 Histologic findings in Sezary syndrome (H&E, 10×) include minimal parakeratosis and spongiosis in a mildly acanthotic epidermis. Note only occasional epidermotropic lymphocytes and a dermal infiltrate of lymphocytes, histiocytes, and eosinophils.

REFERENCES

1. Guitart, J. et al. Histologic criteria for the diagnosis of mycosis fungoides: proposal for a grading system to standardize pathology reporting. *J. Cutan. Pathol.* 28, 174, 2001.
2. Flaxman, B.A., Zelazny, G., and Van Scott, E.J. Non-specificity of characteristic cells in mycosis fungoides. *Arch. Dermatol.* 104, 141, 1971.
3. Everett, M.A. Early diagnosis of mycosis fungoides: vacuolar interface dermatitis. *J. Cutan. Pathol.* 12, 271, 1985.
4. Nickoloff, B.J. Light-microscopic assessment of 100 patients with patch/plaque stage mycosis fungoides. *Am. J. Dermatopathol.* 10, 469, 1988.
5. Lefeber, W.P. et al. Attempts to enhance light microscopic diagnosis of cutaneous T-cell lymphoma (mycosis fungoides). *Arch. Dermatol.* 117, 408, 1981.
6. Olerud, J.E. et al. Cutaneous T-cell lymphoma: evaluation of pretreatment skin biopsy specimens by a panel of pathologists. *Arch. Dermatol.* 128, 501, 1992.
7. Sanchez, J.L. and Ackerman, A.B. The patch stage of mycosis fungoides. *Am. J. Dermatopathol.* 1, 5, 1979.
8. Shapiro, P.E. and Pinto, F.J. The histologic spectrum of mycosis fungoides. Sezary syndrome (cutaneous T-cell lymphoma). A review of 222 biopsies, including newly described patterns and the earliest pathologic changes. *Am. J. Surg. Path.* 18, 645, 1994.
9. Smith, N.P. Histologic criteria for early diagnosis of cutaneous T-cell lymphoma. *Dermatolog. Clin.* 12, 315, 1994.
10. Smoller, B.R. et al. Reassessment of histologic parameters in the diagnosis of mycosis

11. Smoller, B.R. Differentiating early lesions of mycosis fungoides from spongiotic dermatoses. *Pathol. Case Rev.* 1, 158, 1996.
12. McNutt, N.S. and Crain, W.R. Quantitative electron microscopic comparision of lymphocyte nuclear contours in mycosis fungoides and in benign infiltrates in skin. *Cancer* 47, 698, 1981.
13. Lutzner, M.A. et al. Cutaneous T-cell lymphomas: The Sezary syndrome, mycosis fungoides, and related disorders. *Ann. Int. Med.* 83, 534, 1975.
14. Ackerman, A.B. and Flaxman, B.A. Granulomatous mycosis fungoides. *Br. J. Dermatol.* 82, 397, 1970.
15. Smoller, B.R. et al. Role of histology in prognostic information in mycosis fungoides. *J. Cut. Pathol.* 25, 311, 1998.
16. Guitart, J. et al. Lichenoid changes in mycosis fungoides. *J. Am. Acad. Dermatol.* 36, 417, 1997.
17. Vonderbeid, E.C. et al. Clinical implications of immunologic phenotyping in cutaneous T cell lymphoma. *J. Am. Acad. Dermatol.* 17, 40, 1987.
18. Santucci, M. et al. Accuracy, concordance, and reproducibility of histologic diagnosis in cutaneous T-cell lymphoma. *Arch. Dermatol.* 136, 497, 2000.
19. Santucci, M. et al. Cytotoxic/natural killer cell cutaneous lymphomas. Report of EORTC Cutaneous Lymphoma Task Force Workshop. *Cancer* 97, 610, 2003.
20. Ralfkiaer, E. Immunohistochemical markers for the diagnosis of mycosis fungoides. *Semin. Diagn. Pathol.* 8, 61, 1991.
21. Fivenson, D., Hanson, C., and Nickoloff, B. Localization of clonal T-cells to the epidermis in cutaneous T-cell lymphomas. *J. Am. Acad. Dermatol.* 31, 717, 1994.
22. Nickoloff, B.J. Epidermal mucinosis in mycosis fungoides. *J. Am. Acad. Dermatol.* 15, 83, 1996.
23. Diamandidou, E. et al. Transformation of mycosis fungoides/Sezary syndrome: clinical characteristics and prognosis. *Blood* 92, 1150, 1998.
24. Salhany, K.E. et al. Transformation of cutaneous T-cell lymphoma to large cell lymphoma: A clinicopathologic and immunologic study. *Am. J. Pathol.* 132, 265, 1988.
25. van Doorn, R., Scheffer, E., and Willemze, R. Follicular mycosis fungoides, a distinct disease entity with or without associated follicular mucinosis. *Arch. Dermatol.* 138, 191, 2002.
26. Aloi, F., Tomasini, C., and Pippione, M. Mycosis fungoides and eruptive epidermoid cysts: a unique response of follicular and eccrine structures. *Dermatology* 187, 273, 1993.
27. Kossard, S., White, A., and Killingsworth, M. Basaloid folliculolymphoid hyperplasia with alopecia as an expression of mycosis fungoides (CTCL). *J. Cutan. Pathol.* 22, 466, 1995.
28. Flaig, M.J. et al. Follicular mycosis fungoides: A histopathologic analysis of nine cases. *J. Cutan. Pathol.* 28, 525, 2001.
29. Beylot-Barry, M., and Vergier, B. Pilotropic mycosis fungoides. *J. Am. Acad. Dermatol.* 38, 501, 1998.
30. Lacour, J.P. et al. Follicular mycosis fungoides. A clinical and histologic variant of cutaneous T-cell lymphoma: a report of two cases. *J. Am. Acad. Dermatol.* 29, 330, 1993.
31. Pinkus, H. The relationship of alopecia mucinosa to malignant lymphoma. *Dermatologica.* 124, 266, 1964.
32. Zelger, B. et al. Syringotropic cutaneous T-cell lymphoma: a variant of mycosis fungoides? *Br. J. Dermatol.* 130, 765, 1993.

33. Hitchcock, M.G. et al. Eccrine gland infiltration by mycosis fungoides. *Am. J. Dermatopathol.* 18, 447, 1996.
34. Hokak, E. et al. Follicular cutaneous T-cell lymphoma: a clinicopathological study of nine cases. *Br. J. Dermatol.* 141, 315, 1999.
35. Cerroni, L. et al. Follicular mucinosis: a critical approach of clinicopathologic features and association with mycosis fungoides and Sezary syndrome. *Arch Dermatol.* 138, 182, 2002.
36. Wilkinson, J.D., Black, M.M., and Chu, A. Follicular mucinosis associated with mycosis fungoides presenting with gross cystic changes on the face. *Clin. Exp. Dermatol.* 7, 333, 1982.
37. Gibson, L.E. et al. Follicular mucinosis: clinical and histopathologic study. *J. Am. Acad. Dermatol.* 20, 441, 1989.
38. Nickoloff, B.J. and Wood, C. Benign idiopathic versus mycosis-fungoides-associated follicular mucinosis. *Pediatr. Dermatol.* 2, 201, 1985.
39. Cerroni, L. Follicular mucinosis: a critical reappraisal of clinicopathologic features and association with mycosis fungoides and Sezary syndrome. *Arch. Dermatol.* 138, 182, 2002.
40. El-Shabrawi-Caelen, L. et al. Hypopigmented mycosis fungoides: frequent expression of a CD8+ T-cell phenotype. *Am. J. Surg. Pathol.* 26, 450, 2002.
41. Whitmore, S.E., Simmons-O'Brien, E., and Rotter, F.S. Hypopigmented mycosis fungoides. *Arch. Dermatol.* 32, 987, 1995.
42. Lambroza, E. et al. Hypopigmented variant of mycosis fungoides: Demography, histopathology, and treatment of seven cases. *J. Am. Acad. Dermatol.* 32, 987, 1995.
43. Zackheim, H.S. et al. Mycosis fungoides presenting as areas of hypopigmentation. *J. Am. Acad. Dermatol.* 6, 340, 1982.
44. LeBoit, P.E., Zachheim, H.S., and White, C.R. Granulomatous variants of cutaneous T-cell lymphoma. The histopathology of granulomatous mycosis fungoides and granulomatous slack skin. *Am. J. Surg. Pathol.* 12, 83, 1988.
45. LeBoit, P.E. Variants of mycosis fungoides and related cutaneous T-cell lymphomas. *Semin. Diagn. Pathol.* 8, 73, 1991.
46 Mainguene, C. et al. An unusual case of mycosis fungoides presenting as sarcoidosis or granulomatous mycosis fungoides. *Am. J. Clin. Pathol.* 99, 82, 1993.
47. Argenyi, Z.B. et al. Granulomatous mycosis fungoides. Clinicopathologic study of two cases. *Am. J. Dermatopathol.* 18, 199, 1996.
48. Balus, L. Granulomatous slack skin. Report of a case and review of the literature. *Am. J. Dermatopathol.* 14, 200, 1996.
49. Su, L.D. et al. Interstitial mycosis fungoides, a variant of mycosis fungoides resembling granuloma annulare and inflammatory morphea. *J. Cutan. Pathol.* 29, 135, 2002.
50. Lambert, W.C., and Everett, M.A. The nosology of parapsoriasis. *J. Am. Acad. Dermatol.* 5, 373, 1981.
51. Lindae, M.L. et al. Poikilodermatous mycosis fungoides and atrophic large-plaque parapsoriasis exhibit similar abnormalities of T-cell antigen expression. *Arch. Dermatol.* 124, 366, 1988.
52. Kohler, S., Kim, Y.H. and Smoller, B.R. Histologic criteria for the diagnosis of erythrodermic mycosis fungoides and Sezary syndrome: a critical reappraisal. *J. Cutan. Pathol.* 24, 292, 1997.
53. Vonderheid, E.C. et al. Update on erythrodermic cutaneous T-cell lymphoma: report of the International Society for Cutaneous Lymphoma. *J. Am. Acad. Dermatol.* 46, 95, 2002.

54. Buechner, S.A., Winkelmann, R.K. Sézary syndrome. A clinicopathologic study of 39 cases. *Arch. Dermatol.* 119, 979, 1983.
55. Walsh, N.M.G. et al. Histopathology in erythroderma: a review of a series of cases by multiple observers. *J. Cutan. Pathol.* 21, 419, 1994.
56. Winkehnann, R.K. and Linman, J.W. Erythroderma and atypical lymphocytes (Sézary syndrome). *Am. J. Med.* 55, 192, 1973.

4 Sezary Syndrome

Herschel S. Zackheim

CONTENTS

4.1 DEFINITION OF SEZARY SYNDROME

For many years the definition of Sezary syndrome has been unsettled. Clinically, Sezary syndrome is indistinguishable from erythrodermic mycosis fungoides (MF). The decision as to whether the patient has erythrodermic MF or Sezary syndrome depends on whether or not the blood is involved by the neoplastic process. If there is positive evidence of blood involvement, the patient is considered to have Sezary syndrome. If the evidence is not conclusive, a diagnosis of erythrodermic MF is made.

At a meeting of the International Society for Cutaneous Lymphomas (ISCL)[1] blood involvement was defined as the finding of any one or more of the following: (1) an absolute Sezary cell count of 1000 cells/mm³, (2) a CD4/CD8 ratio of 10 caused by an increase in circulating T cells and/or an aberrant loss or expression of pan-T-cell markers by flow cytometry, (3) increased lymphocyte counts with evidence of a T-cell clone in the blood by the Southern blot or polymerase chain reaction technique, or (4) a chromosomally abnormal T-cell clone.

However, recently Vonderheid and Bernengo[2] have critiqued the ISCL definition of Sezary syndrome. Further studies are needed.

4.2 EPIDEMIOLOGY

Substantial numbers of patients with the erythrodermic form of cutaneous T-cell lymphoma (CTCL) have been reported from three institutions. At the University of Graz[3] 281 patients had MF and 22 (7.3%) were stated to have Sezary syndrome. At the University of California, San Francisco (UCSF),[4] 69 of 489 patients (14.1%) with CTCL had erythroderma, otherwise not defined. At Stanford University 15%

of 525 patients with CTCL had erythroderma, also not otherwise defined.[5] These data provide only an approximation of the frequency of Sezary syndrome because the definition of Sezary syndrome at Graz may differ from the recently adopted definition by the ISCL,[1] and the UCSF and Stanford data were based on erythroderma only and not on other criteria for Sezary syndrome.

The erythrodermic form of CTCL involves the oldest age group of CTCL patients. Of 489 patients with CTCL seen at UCSF in the past 50 years or more, the mean age of the erythrodermic patients was 64.2 years as compared to a mean age of 59.4, 56.9, and 52.3 years for patients with tumor-stage (T3), extensive patch/plaque (T2), and limited extent patch/plaque disease (T1), respectively.[4] Similarly, in the Stanford cohort of 525 CTCL patients,[5] the median age of patients with erythrodermic CTCL was 65 years and that for stages T3, T2, and T1 was 58, 58, and 49 years, respectively.

4.3 CLINICAL FEATURES

The clinical features of Sezary syndrome are indistinguishable from those described for erythrodermic MF. (See chapter 2.)

4.4 HISTOPATHOLOGY

Trotter et al.[6] evaluated skin biopsies in 41 erythrodermic patients with circulating Sezary cells and a clonal population of T cells detected by T-cell receptor-gene rearrangement on Southern blot analysis of peripheral blood mononuclear cells. Histopathologic features consistent with chronic dermatitis were observed in 33% of the biopsies, demonstrating that a nonspecific histology is common in patients with Sezary syndrome.

4.5 TREATMENT

Winkelmann et al.[7] introduced the use of continuous low-dose chlorambucil and predisolone for Sezary syndrome, and this has been widely used since. The principal risks are bone marrow depression and secondary leukemia. More recently Coors and von den Driesch[8] obtained favorable results with intermittent chlorambucil and fluocortolone in erythrodermic CTCL. Zackheim et al.[9] obtained a beneficial outcome in 29 patients with erythrodermic CTCL treated with low-dose methotrexate. The total response rate was 58%. The median period from start of treatment to treatment failure was 31 months, and the median overall survival was 8.4 years. Side effects caused treatment failure in only 2 patients.

Extracorporeal photochemotherapy (ECP) for erythrodermic CTCL was first reported by Edelson et al. in 1987[10] and is widely used for that condition. Nevertheless, the value of ECP as a single agent for Sezary syndrome remains controversial. Fraser-Andrews et al.[11] found no significant effect on the survival of 44 patients with a peripheral blood T-cell clone. There have been a considerable number of but few relating to ECP therapy as a single agent. Of note is the report from the Mayo Clinic[12] that only 1 of 55 patients with Sezary syndrome treated with ECP alone achieved a sustained remission.

Forty-five patients with erythrodermic MF were treated at McMaster University, Ontario, and at Yale University with total skin electron beam therapy [13] as a single modality. The rate of complete cutaneous remission was 60%, with 26% remaining progression free at 5 years.

Interferon-alfa has demonstrated activity against Sezary syndrome, although the response rate is not high. The largest series of Sezary syndrome patients treated with interferon-alfa as monotherapy was reported by Jumbou et al.[14] Of 11 patients, 2 achieved complete remission, 1 partial remission, and 8 stable or progressive disease.

This author has managed two patients with Sezary syndrome who failed methotrexate and remained clear for over 1 year with interferon-alfa therapy (Zackheim, unpublished).

Rosen and Foss[15] reviewed chemotherapy for CTCL as of 1995. They concluded that there are no studies that clearly demonstrate improvement of survival.

Bouwhuis et al.[16] reviewed records of 6 patients with Sezary syndrome who had been treated with 2-chlorodeoxyadenosine (2-CdA). Two responded well; 4 had only a partial or no response. The mortality rate was 50%. All 3 patients died of *Staphylococcus aureus* sepsis.

Lundin et al.[17] obtained an overall response rate of 69% in patients with erythroderma treated with alemtuzumab (anti-CD52 monoclonal antibody). Fierro et al.[18] failed to obtain responses in 2 patients with Sezary syndrome treated with combination etoposide, idarubicin, cyclophosphamide, vincristine, prednisone, and bleomycin (VICOP-B). Scarisbrick et al.[19] treated 8 patients with Sezary syndrome with combination fludarabine and cyclophosphamide; of these 5 had a response. The mean duration of response was 10 months. Six of the patients failed treatment, 5 due to bone marrow depression and 1 due to progressive disease.

Denileukin diftitox is a relatively new addition to the list of agents that are active against resistant or advanced-stage CTCL.[20] It is a novel recombinant fusion protein consisting of domains of diphtheria toxin and human interleukin (IL)-2. Two of 6 patients with erythroderma treated with a dose level of 18 μg/kg/d achieved a partial response. Constitutional and gastrointestinal symptoms were the most common side effects. At least one symptom affected 92% of the patients. The vascular leak syndrome occurred in 25% of the patients and was usually self-limited.

Bexarotene (Targretin) is a novel retinoid (rexinoid) that is FDA-approved for the treatment of CTCL. In a multi-institutional study[21] responses were obtained in 6 of 19 patients (32%) with erythroderma. Four of 17 patients (24%) with Sezary syndrome responded. The principal side effects were hyperlipemia, pruritus, and hypothyroidism. High triglyceride or cholesterol levels occurred within 2 to 4 weeks after start of therapy. One patient developed serious but reversible pancreatitis.

Talpur et al.[22] confirmed the overall effectiveness of bexarotene in CTCL in a single institution study; however, responses for erythrodermic MF or Sezary syndrome as single entities were not presented. The authors stated that the use of statins may increase the response rates with acceptable toxicity risk, but data in this regard

TABLE 4.1
Survival Data for Erythrodermic Cutaneous T-Cell Lymphoma

Institution and Year	No. of Sezary Patients	No. of Stage T4 Patients	5-Year Survival (%)		10-Year Survival (%)		Ref.
			Overall	Disease Specific	Overall	Disease Specific	
Spain (four centers), 2003	29	N/A	38	N/A	N/A	N/A	24
Stanford, 2003	N/A	78	41	65	24	N/A	5
Graz, 2002	22	N/A	33	N/A	N/A	N/A	3
UCSF, 1999	N/A	69	51	N/A	30	N/A	4
Turin, 1998	62	N/A	33	N/A	N/A	N/A	23

Note: UCSF, University of California, San Francisco.

4.6 PROGNOSIS

Table 4.1 presents long-term survival data for erythrodermic CTCL from five medical centers (the report from Spain combines four centers) with substantial numbers of such patients. For generalized erythroderma (stage T4, not otherwise defined) 5-year overall survival rates for Stanford and UCSF were 41% and 51%, respectively; the corresponding 10-year survival rates were 24% and 30%. Both the University of Graz[2] and the University of Turin[23] had a 5-year survival rate of 33%, and the combined results from four dermatology departments in Spain revealed a 5-year survival rate of 38%.[24]

REFERENCES

1. Vonderheid, E.C. et al. Update on erythrodermic cutaneous T-cell lymphoma: Report of the International Society for Cutaneous Lymphomas. *J. Am. Acad. Dermatol.* 46, 95, 2002.
2. Vonderheid, E.C. and Bernengo, M.G. The Sezary syndrome: hematologic criteria. *Hematol. Oncol. Clin. N. Amer.* 17, 1367, 2003.
3. Fink-Puches, R. et al. Primary cutaneous lymphomas: applicability of current classification schemes (European Organization for Research and Treatment of Cancer, World Health Organization) based on clinicopathologic features observed in a large group of patients. *Blood* 99, 800, 2002.
4. Zackheim, H.S. et al. Prognosis in cutaneous T-cell lymphoma by skin type: Long-term survival in 489 patients. *J. Am. Acad. Dermatol.* 40, 418, 1999.
5. Kim, Y.H. et al. Long-term outcome of 525 patients with mycosis fungoides and Sezary syndrome. *Arch. Dermatol.* 139, 857, 2003.
6. Trotter, M.J. et al. Cutaneous histopathology of Sezary syndrome: a study of 41 cases with a proven circulating T-cell clone. *J. Cutan. Pathol.* 24, 286, 1997.
7. Winkelmann, R., Diaz-Perez, H., and Buechner, S. The treatment of Sezary syndrome.

8. Coors, E.A. and von den Driesch, P. Treatment of erythrodermic cutaneous T-cell lymphoma with intermittent chlorambucil and fluocortolone therapy. *Br. J. Dermatol.* 143, 127, 2000.

9. Zackheim, H.S., Kashani-Sabet, M., and Amin, S. Low-dose methotrexate to treat erythrodermic cutaneous T-cell lymphoma: Results in twenty-nine patients. *J. Am. Acad. Dermatol.* 34, 626, 1996.

10. Edelson, R. et al. Treatment of cutaneous T-cell lymphoma by extracorporeal photochemotherapy. *New England J. Med.* 316, 297, 1987.

11. Fraser-Andrews, E. et al. Extracorporeal photopheresis in Sezary syndrome. No significant effect in the survival of 44 patients with a peripheral blood T-cell clone. *Arch. Dermatol.* 134, 1001, 1998.

12. Bouwhuis, S.A., McEvoy, M.T., and Davis, M.D. Sustained remission of Sezary syndrome. *Eur. J. Dermatol.* 12, 287, 2002.

13. Jones, G.W., Rosenthal, D., and Wilson, L.D. Total skin electron radiation for patients with erythrodermic cutaneous T-cell lymphoma (mycosis fungoides and the Sezary syndrome). *Cancer* 85, 1985, 1999.

14. Jumbou, O. et al. Long-term follow-up in 51 patients with mycosis fungoides and Sezary syndrome treated by interferon-alfa. *Br. J. Dermatol.* 140, 427, 1999.

15. Rosen, S.T. and Foss, F.M. Chemotherapy for mycosis fungoides and the Sezary syndrome. *Hematol./Oncol. Clin. North Am.* 9, 1109, 1995.

16. Bouwhuis, S.A. et al. Treatment of late-stage Sezary syndrome with 2-chlorodeoxyadenosine. *Int. J. Dermatol.* 41, 352, 2002.

17. Lundin, J. et al. Phase 2 study of alemtuzumab (anti-CD52 monoclonal antibody) in patients with advanced mycosis fungoides/Sezary syndrome. *Blood* 101, 4267, 2003.

18. Fierro, M.T. et al. Combination of etoposide, idarubicin, cyclophosphamide, vincristine, prednisone and bleomycin (VICOP-B) in the treatment of advanced cutaneous T-cell lymphoma. *Dermatology* 194, 268, 1997.

19. Scarisbrick, J.J. et al. A trial of fludarabine and cyclophosphamide combination chemotherapy in the treatment of advanced refractory primary cutaneous T-cell lymphoma. *Br. J. Dermatol.* 144, 1010, 2001.

20. Olsen, E. et al. Pivotal phase III trial of two dose levels of denileukin diftitox for the treatment of cutaneous T-cell lymphoma. *J. Clin. Oncol.* 19, 376, 2001.

21. Duvic, M. et al. Bexarotene is effective and safe for treatment of refractory advanced-stage cutaneous T-cell lymphoma: multinational phase II–III trial results. *J. Clin. Oncol.* 19, 2456, 2001.

22. Talpur, R. et al. Optimizing bexarotene therapy for cutaneous T-cell lymphoma. *J. Am. Acad. Dermatol.* 47, 672, 2002.

23. Bernengo, M.G. et al. Prognostic factors in Sezary syndrome: a multivariate analysis of clinical, haematological and immunological features. *Ann. Oncol.* 9, 857, 1998.

24. Marti, R.M. et al. Sezary syndrome and related variants of classic cutaneous T-cell lymphoma. A descriptive and prognostic clinicopathologic study of 29 cases. *Leuk. Lymphoma* 44, 59, 2003.

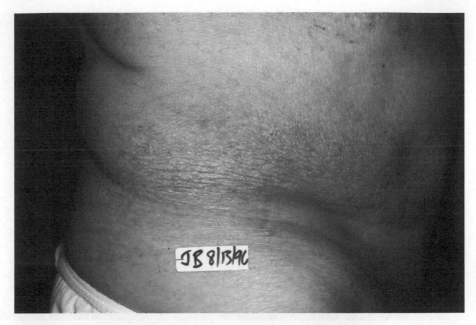

COLOR FIGURE 2.1 Patch-stage mycosis fungoides on the lower flank.

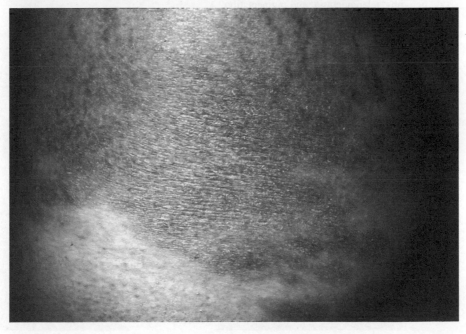

COLOR FIGURE 2.2 Patch-stage mycosis fungoides on the lateral buttocks.

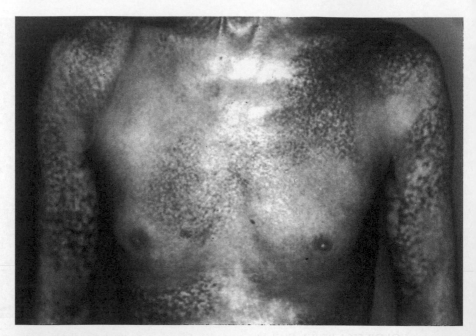

COLOR FIGURE 2.4 Almost universal poikilodermatous mycosis fungoides. There is atrophy, telangiectasia, and pigmentation.

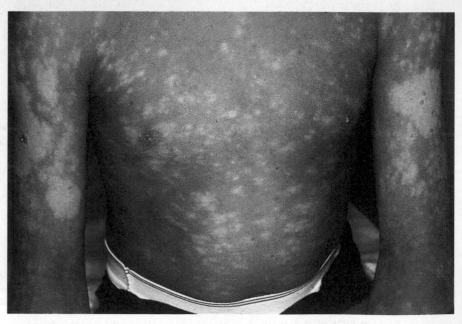

COLOR FIGURE 2.6 Extensive hypopigmented mycosis fungoides.

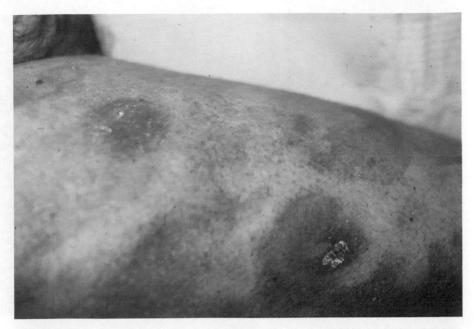

COLOR FIGURE 2.8 Multiple lesions of plaque-stage mycosis fungoides on the thigh.

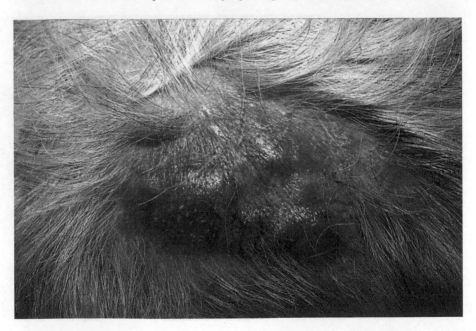

COLOR FIGURE 2.10 Nodules of tumor-stage mycosis fungoides on the scalp.

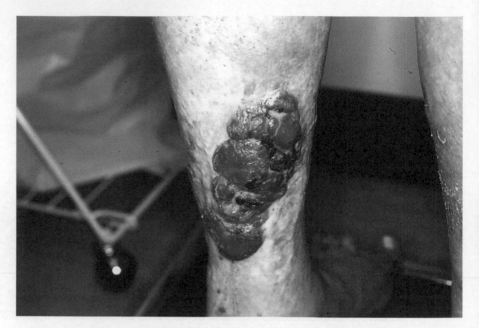

COLOR FIGURE 2.12 Exuberant mycosis fungoides tumor on the leg.

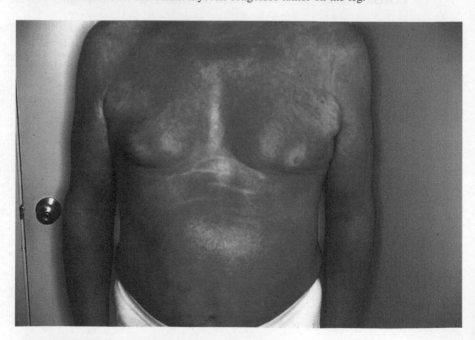

COLOR FIGURE 2.13 Universal erythroderma.

5 Lymphomatoid Papulosis

Herschel S. Zackheim and Bruce R. Smoller

CONTENTS

5.1 EPIDEMIOLOGY

Lymphomatoid papulosis (LyP) involves a somewhat younger age group than the more common form of cutaneous T-cell lymphoma (CTCL) mycosis fungoides (MF). The median age of 118 LyP patients in the Dutch group was 45.5 years[1] as compared to a mean age of 55.9 years (median age not stated) at diagnosis in 174 MF patients reported by Whittemore et al.[2] LyP is well documented in children.[3] As with MF, LyP tends to be more common in males than females. In the Dutch group the male to female ratio was 1.4. No causative factors have been established.

5.2 CLINICAL FEATURES

The indispensable clinical feature permitting a diagnosis of LyP is the occurrence of self-involuting papules. Often a histologic diagnosis of "consistent with" or "suggestive of" LyP is made. However, unless there is unequivocal clinical evidence of a self-involuting papular eruption, a diagnosis of LyP cannot be made.

The typical LyP lesion is a 3 to 5 mm red papule with a central crust (Figures 5.1 and 5.2). In some patients the crusted papules are somewhat larger than 5 mm (Figure 5.3) in which case differentiation from anaplastic large cell lymphoma (ALCL) may be difficult, or they may be only 1 to 2 mm in diameter without obvious crusting (Figure 5.4). LyP lesions are usually widely scattered and typically present in different stages of evolution (Figure 5.5). However, they may have only a regional

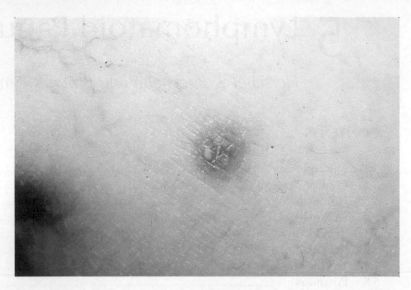

FIGURE 5.1 Close view of lymphomatoid papulosis papule shows an inflammatory lesion with a central crust.

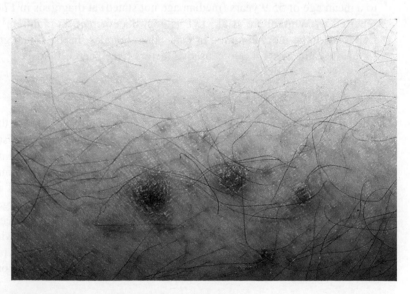

FIGURE 5.2 Multiple lymphomatoid papulosis papules.

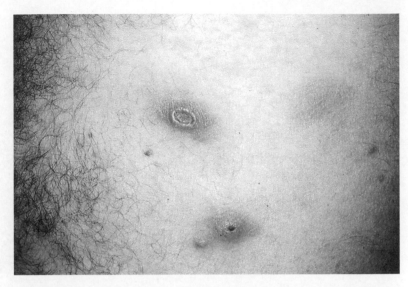

FIGURE 5.3 Crusted lymphomatoid papulosis papules (LyP) are larger than average and are eroded. Differentiation from anaplastic large cell lymphoma is difficult, but histology favored LyP.

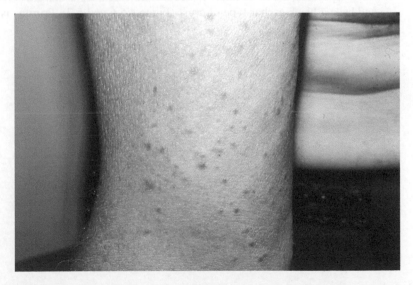

FIGURE 5.4 Lymphomatoid papulosis (LyP) papules are only 1 to 2 mm in diameter; however, histology was definite for LyP. Additionally, the lesions were limited to the leg.

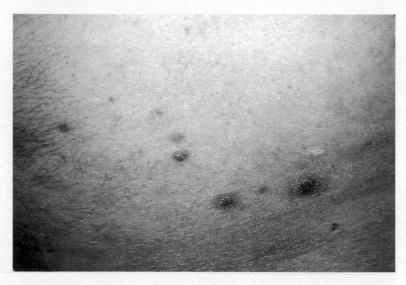

FIGURE 5.5 Multiple papules of lymphomatoid papulosis on abdomen in different stages of evolution. The lesions were widely distributed over the body surface.

distribution (Figure 5.4); this occurred in 13% of the 118 patients with LyP in the Dutch group.[1]

LyP lesions involute predominantly without scar formation (contrary to the literature); however, in a small proportion of cases a scar follows. Scars, which are often depressed, are more likely to occur following lesions that are severely inflamed and have a black eschar type of crust (Figures 5.6 and 5.7). Pruritus is usually mild

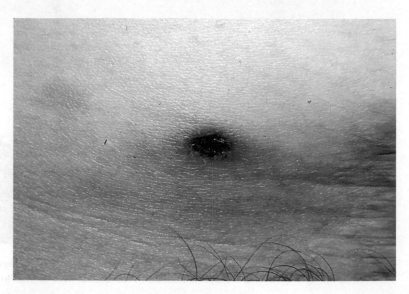

FIGURE 5.6 Severely inflamed papule with black eschar.

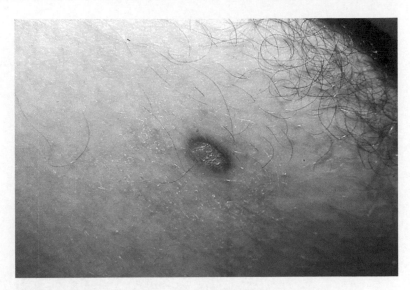

FIGURE 5.7 Papule shown in Figure 5.6 resolved leaving a depressed scar.

or absent in LyP but may be bothersome in some patients. LyP is predominantly a chronic disorder. In 50% of patients with LyP the disease persisted for more than 10 years.[4]

5.3 HISTOPATHOLOGY

Three different histologic patterns have been described in patients with LyP.[5] The most common, and most characteristic, is subtype A. In these biopsies the unique feature is the presence of large, atypical dermal lymphocytes that resemble the Reed–Sternberg cells of Hodgkin's lymphoma (Figures 5.8 and 5.9). The cells have eosinophilic cytoplasm and vesicular nuclei with prominent eosinophilic nucleoli. There may be multiple nucleoli present within single cells and multinucleated forms are also present. These atypical cells demonstrate mitotic activity, and individual cell necrosis is common. The atypical cells represent only a minority of the dermal infiltrate, usually on the order of 20% to 30% of the dermal inflammatory cellular population.

Less common is the subtype B LyP. These biopsies are characterized by an infiltrate of enlarged, hyperconvoluted and hyperchromatic lymphocytes that resemble the cells seen in MF (Figure 5.10). These atypical lymphocytes again represent only a minority of the dermal cellular infiltrate and are admixed with the reactive lymphocytes and scattered eosinophils. There is a greater tendency for epidermotropism with this subtype than is seen in subtype A.

The final histologic subtype of LyP is the relatively newly described subtype C. In these cases the vast majority of the dermal infiltrate is comprised of the Reed–Sternberg-like, atypical lymphocytes. There is a relatively sparse dermal inflammatory response. In addition, the density of the infiltrate is more intense, often

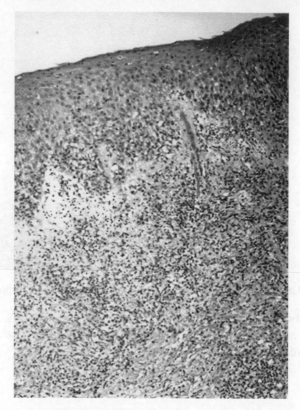

FIGURE 5.8 Low magnification (100×) demonstrates a superficial and deep, dense wedge-shaped infiltrate of hematopoietic cells.

Individual patients may have simultaneous lesions with more than one histologic pattern or have evolving patterns. In addition, some individual biopsies may demonstrate more than one of the described patterns.

The architectural features of LyP are shared by patients with different subtypes.[6] These include a dense, dermal wedge-shaped infiltrate of inflammatory cells that often extends into the overlying epidermis (Figure 5.8).

Spongiosis and parakeratosis are seen in most, but not all cases. Rare dying keratinocytes may be present in the lower portions of the epidermis. The majority of the dermal infiltrate is comprised of small, reactive lymphocytes. Admixed eosinophils are present in most cases. In some cases, neutrophils may be present within and around vessel walls, giving an appearance similar to a focal leukocytoclastic vasculitis. The dermal infiltrate is centered around blood vessels; blood is often extensive enough to extend into the surrounding interstitial collagen. Perifollicular involvement has been described but is not present in all cases. Extension into the subcutaneous fat is not a common finding.

Lymphocyte immunophenotyping plays a role in arriving at a biopsy diagnosis of LyP.[7] In all cases the dermal infiltrate is comprised of CD3+ T lymphocytes. The small reactive T cells demonstrate a CD4 predominance over CD8+ cells.[8] Only rare

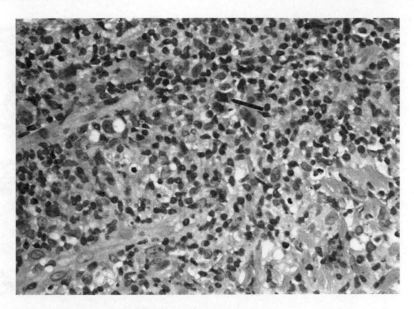

FIGURE 5.9 Type A cells resemble Reed–Sternberg cells in having enlarged vesicular nuclei, prominent nucleoli, and abundant cytoplasm (200×).

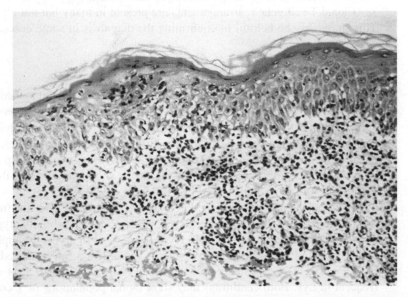

FIGURE 5.10 In type B lymphomatoid papulosis there is an infiltrate of hyperchromatic and hyperconvoluted lymphocytes that demonstrate extensive epidermotropism (100×).

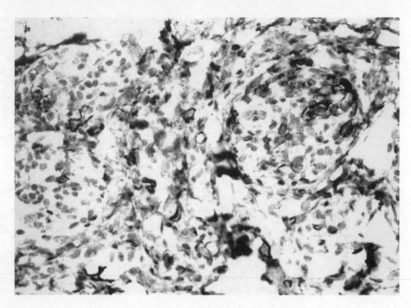

FIGURE 5.11 The atypical cells in type A lymphomatoid papulosis strongly express CD30 (200×).

B cells are seen. The large atypical cells may express CD4, or in some cases may fail to express the common pan-T-cell surface antigens. In subtypes A and C, CD30 is strongly expressed by the large atypical cells. This is the most specific immunostain for arriving at the diagnosis. CD25 may be expressed by these cells.

Clonal T-cell gene rearrangements are present in many but not all cases of LyP. This study may be helpful in confirming the diagnosis in some cases.[9-11]

5.4 DIFFERENTIAL DIAGNOSIS

The principal disorder from which LyP needs to be distinguished is pityriasis lichenoides et varioliformis acuta (PLEVA),[4] and for many years there was controversy as to whether LyP and PLEVA were the same or different conditions.

Both entities are characterized by recurrent inflammatory papules, but these are usually smaller and more numerous in PLEVA. A younger age group is more often involved in PLEVA. The duration of disease is shorter in PLEVA than in LyP: 6 months in 30% of patients with PLEVA versus only 4% in LyP.

Histologically, eosinophils and perivascular neutrophils are not frequently seen in PLEVA. Further, and more specifically, while occasional slightly atypical lymphocytes may populate the dermis in PLEVA, the number of atypical lymphocytes is not that seen in LyP. CD30 is not expressed by more than a few scattered lymphocytes in PLEVA. CD8+ cells usually predominate in PLEVA, whereas CD4+ cells are more frequent in LyP. Both conditions may show clonal populations of T cells.

The histologic differential diagnosis also includes Hodgkin's disease, MF, ALCL, and perhaps arthropod bite reaction in some cases.[12-13] Long-standing arthropod bite reactions may demonstrate rare atypical cells that may even express CD30, but they do not constitute a significant percentage of the dermal inflammatory infiltrate. In contrast, cutaneous Hodgkin's disease and ALCL are characterized by dermal cellular infiltrates with many atypical lymphocytes. In ALCL the vast majority of cells are atypical and express CD30. This atypical population is much in excess of that seen in LyP (except for subtype C, which may represent the same disease). In Hodgkin's disease the distinction must be made based on clinical distinction and the other histologic features such as fibrosis, nodular configurations to the infiltrate, and lacunar cells not seen in LyP. It can be virtually impossible to distinguish type B LyP from MF. In these situations clinical history is probably the best discriminator.

5.5 RELATION TO CD30+ ALCL

LyP and ALCL are generally considered to be part of the spectrum of CD30+ lymphoproliferative disorders. Overall, LyP is a benign disorder, whereas ALCL is recognized as a true lymphoma although it generally behaves in a more benign manner than most other lymphomas (see chapter 6).

5.6 RELATION TO LYMPHOMAS OTHER THAN ALCL

MF has been found in patients with LyP in a number of studies. In a very recent study from the University of California, San Francisco (UCSF),[11] MF was found in 21 of 54 patients (39%) with LyP. This is the highest association yet to be recorded. In the same report[11] in a literature review that included 5 series involving at least 40 patients each, MF was associated with LyP in 7% to 18% of the patients.

5.7 TREATMENT

The great majority of LyP patients do not require treatment for the following reasons: (a) LyP is predominantly a benign disorder; (b) none of the recognized treatments for LyP, most importantly low-dose methotrexate,[14] have an effect on the long-term course of the disease; and (c) as a rule, LyP patients are asymptomatic or only mildly symptomatic.

At UCSF methotrexate, usually in oral doses of 5 to 20 mg once weekly, is used primarily in patients who (a) are symptomatic, usually due to pruritus; (b) develop scarring lesions; and (c) develop lesions in cosmetically sensitive areas, such as the face. We have also found topical clobetasol and topical carmustine[15] to be helpful in some patients.

5.8 PROGNOSIS

LyP is predominantly a benign, chronic disorder. The overall prognosis for long-term survival in LyP patients is excellent. The 5- and 10-year disease-related survival in the Dutch group was 100%.[1]

REFERENCES

1. Bekkenk, M.W. et al. Primary and secondary cutaneous CD30+ lymphoproliferative disorders: a report from the Dutch Cutaneous Lymphoma Group on the long-term follow-up data of 219 patients and guidelines for diagnosis and treatment. *Blood* 95, 3653, 2000.
2. Whittemore, A.S. Mycosis fungoides in relation to environmental exposures and immune response: a case-control study. *J. Natl. Cancer Inst.* 81, 1560, 1989.
3. Van Neer, F.J.M.A. et al. Lymphomatoid papulosis in children: a study of 10 children registered by the Dutch Cutaneous Lymphoma Working Group. *Br. J. Dermatol.* 144, 351, 2001.
4. Willemze, R. and Scheffer, E. Clinical and histologic differentiation between lymphomatoid papulosis and pityriasis lichenoides. *J. Am. Acad. Dermatol.* 13, 418, 1985.
5. Drews, R., Samel, A., and Kadin, M.E. Lymphomatoid papulosis and anaplastic large cell lymphomas of the skin. *Semin. Cutaneous Med. Surg.* 19, 109, 2000.
6. Karp, D.L. and Horn, T.D. Lymphomatoid papulosis. *J. Am. Acad. Dermatol.* 30, 379, 1994.
7. El-Azhary, R.A. et al. Lymphomatoid papulosis: A clinical and histopathologic review of 53 cases with leukocyte immunophenotyping, DNA flow cytometry, and T-cell receptor gene rearrangement studies. *J. Am. Acad. Dermatol.* 30, 210, 1994.
8. Kadin, M.E. et al. Lymphomatoid papulosis. A cutaneous proliferation of activated helper cells expressing Hodgkin's disease-associated antigen. *Am. J. Pathol.* 119, 315, 1985.
9. Zelickson, B.D. et al. T-cell receptor gene rearrangement analysis: Cutaneous T cell lymphoma, peripheral T cell lymphoma, and premalignant and benign cutaneous lymphoproliferative disorders. *J. Am. Acad. Dermatol.* 25, 787, 1991.
10. Steinhoff, M. et al. Single-cell analysis of CD30+ cells in lymphomatoid papulosis demonstrates a common clonal T-cell origin. *Blood* 100, 578, 2002.
11. Zackheim, H.S. et al. Lymphomatoid papulosis associated with mycosis fungoides: a study of 21 patients including analyses for clonality. *J. Am. Acad. Dermatol.* 49, 620, 2003.
12. Kadin, M.E. Lymphomatoid papulosis, Ki-1+ lymphoma, and primary cutaneous Hodgkin's disease. *Semin. Dermatol.* 10, 164, 1991.
13. Smoller, B.R., Longacre, T.A., and Warnke, R.A. Ki-1 (CD30) expression in differentiation of lymphomatoid papulosis from arthropod bite reactions. *Mod. Pathol.* 5, 492, 1992.
14. Vonderheid, E.C., Sajjadian, A., and Kadin, M.E. Methotrexate is effective therapy for lymphomatoid papulosis and other primary cutaneous CD30-positive lymphoproliferative disorders. *J. Am. Acad. Dermatol.* 34, 470, 1996.
15. Zackheim, H.S., Epstein, E.H., Jr., and Crain, W.R. Topical carmustine therapy for lymphomatoid papulosis. *Arch. Dermatol.* 121, 1410, 1985.

6 Primary Cutaneous CD30+ Anaplastic Large Cell Lymphoma

Herschel S. Zackheim and Bruce R. Smoller

CONTENTS

6.1 EPIDEMIOLOGY

Anaplastic large cell lymphoma (ALCL) involves an older age group than the closely related CD30+ lymphoproliferative disorder lymphomatoid papulosis (LyP). The median age of the 79 patients with ALCL in the Dutch group was 60 years at diagnosis[1] as compared to a median age of 45.5 years for the 118 LyP patients in that cohort.

6.2 CLINICAL FEATURES

Patients with ALCL may present with nodules, papules, or ulcerated, infiltrated lesions (Figures 6.1–6.4). In the Dutch series of 79 patients, 42 patients (53%) presented with a solitary tumor, which may have ulcerated; 20 patients (25%) presented with several grouped nodules or papules restricted to one region. Multi-focal disease (at multiple anatomic sites) was found in 17 patients (22%). A strong tendency for partial or complete spontaneous remission was noted; this occurred in 33 patients (42%).

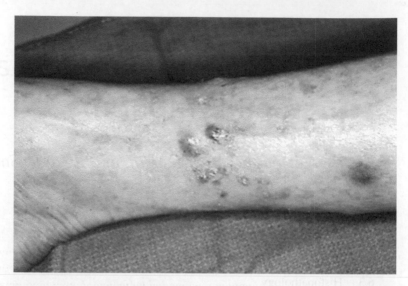

FIGURE 6.1 Nodules and papules of CD30+ anaplastic large cell lymphoma on leg.

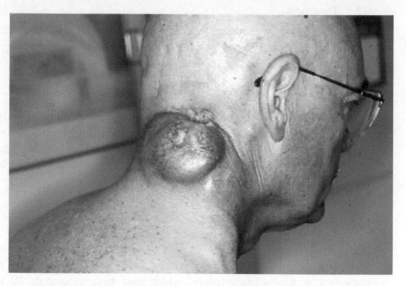

FIGURE 6.2 Huge tumor of CD30+ anaplastic large cell lymphoma on back of neck. There is a small central erosion.

6.3 HISTOPATHOLOGY

ALCL has a characteristic histologic appearance. The epidermis is often compressed by a dense dermal infiltrate of large, cytologically atypical cells. Epidermotropism is usually scant to nonexistent. Some lesions are characterized by ulceration, though extensive epidermal invasion by neoplastic cells is unusual. In some cases a grenz zone may be present within the papillary dermis. The dermis is replete with large

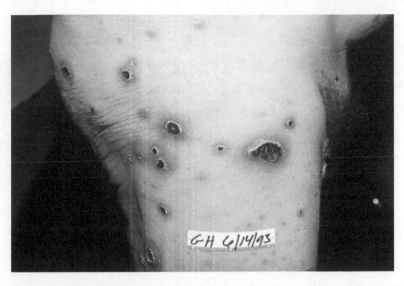

FIGURE 6.3 Multiple infiltrated and erosive lesions of histologically confirmed CD30+ anaplastic large cell lymphoma on the lateral thigh.

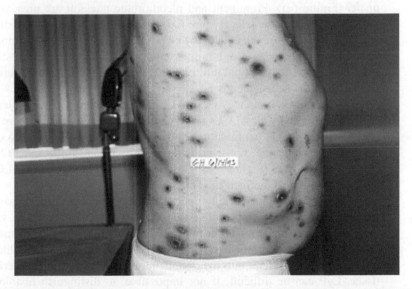

FIGURE 6.4 Extensive lesions of CD30+ anaplastic large cell lymphoma on lateral trunk in same patient shown in Figure 3. The lesions involved all areas of the body. One of the biopsies showed changes that could represent either lymphomatoid papulosis or CD30+ anaplastic large cell lymphoma. This patient illustrates the spectrum of disease of CD30+ lymphoproliferative disorders. He experienced complete remission in about 10 years.

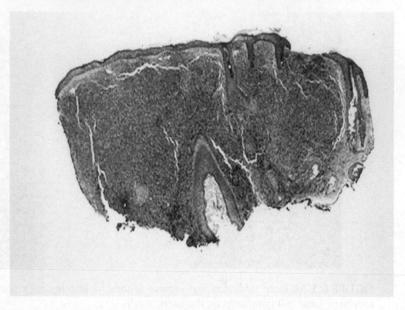

FIGURE 6.5 Low magnification demonstrates diffuse infiltrate of lymphocytes completely filling the dermis.

lymphocytes that have moderate amounts of eosinophilic cytoplasm and vesicular nuclei (Figure 6.5). Prominent and pleomorphic nucleoli are present and may be multiple within single cells (Figure 6.6). Multinucleated cells, including some that resemble Reed–Sternberg cells, may be present. Dense clusters and nodules of cells fill the dermis. There is a high mitotic rate and individual cell necrosis is extensive in many cases. The lymphoid infiltrate diffusely involves the entire dermis and often extends into the subcutaneous fat.

The neoplastic lymphocytes in ALCL have a characteristic pattern of antigen expression. Virtually all ALCLs are T-cell lymphomas; however, there is frequently aberrant loss of CD3 expression. The majority of these tumors also express CD4. The identifying feature, however, is the diffuse expression of CD30 by these neoplastic lymphocytes (Figure 6.7). The neoplastic lymphocytes in ALCL also stain epithelial membrane antigen in some cases.

In contrast to angiocentric lymphomas, the lymphocytes do not have a tendency to invade muscle walls and local infarction is not present. In addition, while involvement of the subcutaneous fat is not uncommon, the tumors are situated primarily within the reticular dermis, in contrast to subcutaneous panniculitis-like T-cell lymphomas that may extend into the dermis but are centered in the underlying adipose tissue. LyP can be difficult, if not impossible, to distinguish histologically from ALCL. Type A LyP is characterized by a dermal infiltrate of large, atypical lymphocytes that are histologically identical to those seen in ALCL. However, in ALCL the vast majority of the dermal infiltrate has this morphologic appearance, while in type A LyP the atypical lymphocytes constitute a minority population. A dense, wedge-shaped infiltrate of reaction T cells admixed with eosinophils and perivascular

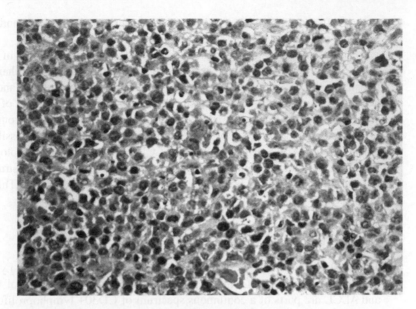

FIGURE 6.6 Higher magnification demonstrates sheets of pleomorphic large lymphocytes with abundant mitotic activity and individual cell necrosis.

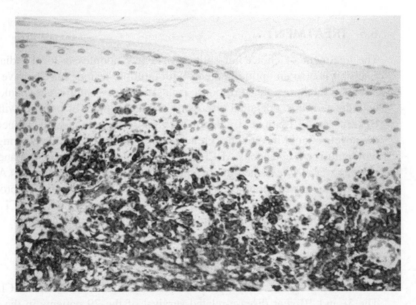

FIGURE 6.7 CD30 expression is demonstrated on the vast majority of lymphocytes in primary cutaneous large cell anaplastic lymphoma.

neutrophils is also present within the dermis. The distinction from type C LyP is more difficult, if not impossible. In this form of the disease, the dermal infiltrate is histologically identical to ALCL in that virtually all of the infiltrating lymphocytes display the atypical cellular characteristics. The distinction is made largely on clinical grounds. It should also be noted that some experts believe ALCL and type C LyP to be the same entity.

Patients with long-standing histories of mycosis fungoides (MF) in whom transformation to tumor stage is occurring will demonstrate histologic changes that are indistinguishable from those seen in ALCL. The hyperconvoluted and hyperchromatic cells and the epidermotropism characteristic of early stages of MF are not seen in advanced disease. In addition, CD30 expression becomes common, unlike in early stage lesions, where it is invariably absent. It is also not possible to distinguish primary ALCL from secondary ALCL based on routine histologic sections. In many cases cutaneous involvement by systemic ALCL will demonstrate anaplastic lymphoma kinase (ALK) positivity and a true T12:15 translocation. This is not seen in primary cutaneous ALCL.

6.4 DIFFERENTIAL DIAGNOSIS

The most difficult distinction is between large papular lesions of LyP and small nodular lesions of ALCL. In fact, the distinction is largely artificial because LyP and ALCL are parts of a continuous spectrum of CD30+ lymphoproliferative disorders. Nodular lesions of ALCL may be difficult to distinguish clinically from tumor stage MF. Differentiation is usually possible on the basis of histology.

6.5 TREATMENT

The treatment of choice for solitary or a few nodules is local radiation therapy. Excision is also an option. Patients with multiple lesions may be given a trial with low-dose methotrexate. If response is unsatisfactory, multiagent chemotherapy may be indicated. For a detailed discussion of management of patients with ALCL, see Bekkenk et al.[1] Keun et al.[2] reported response of a patient with cutaneous ALCL to the novel retinoid bexarotene. French et al.[3] obtained dramatic clearing of a patient with multifocal cutaneous ALCL with combination interferon alfa and bexarotene. Schwartz et al.[4] described improvement in a patient with cutaneous ALCL treated with extracorporeal photochemotherapy. Reinhold et al.[5] obtained prolonged complete remission in a patient with treatment-resistant cutaneous ALCL treated with high-dose chemotherapy and autologous stem cell transplantation.

6.6 PROGNOSIS

The overall prognosis for patients with primary cutaneous CD30+ ALCL is excellent. The 5- and 10-year disease-related survival of the 79 patients in the Dutch group was 96%.[1] Only 4 of the patients (5%) died of lymphoma. Thus, the difference in prognosis between patients with LyP and ALCL is not as great as was believed some years ago. Nevertheless, the calculated risk for extracutaneous disease at 5 and 10 years for patients with ALCL was 9% and 16%, respectively, as compared to 2% and 4% for patients with LyP.

REFERENCES

1. Bekkenk, M.W. et al. Primary and secondary cutaneous CD30+ lymphoproliferative disorders: a report from the Dutch Cutaneous Lymphoma Group on the long-term follow-up data of 219 patients and guidelines for diagnosis and treatment. *Blood* 95, 3653, 2000.
2. Keun, Y.K., Woodruff, R. and Sangueza, O. Response of CD30+ large cell lymphoma of skin to bexarotene. *Leuk. Lymphoma* 43, 1153, 2002.
3. French, L.E. et al. Regression of multifocal, skin-restricted, CD30-positive large T-cell lymphoma with interferon alfa and bexarotene therapy. *J. Am. Acad. Dermatol.* 45, 914, 2001.
4. Schwartz, J. et al. Extracorporeal photochemothrapy in a patient with K-1-positive anaplastic large cell lymphoma. *Br. J. Dermatol.* 134, 332, 1996.
5. Reinhold, U. et al. High-dose chemotherapy with autologous stem cell transplantation in a patient with a CD30+ anaplastic large cell lymphoma of the skin. *Br. J. Dermatol.* 134, 808, 1996.

7 Follicular Mucinosis

Lawrence E. Gibson

CONTENTS

Follicular Mucinosis

Synonyms: Alopecia mucinosa (Pinkus); benign and lymphoma-associated follicular mucinosis (Braun-Falco)[1,2]

ICD9 Code: 704.09

7.1 HISTORICAL PERSPECTIVE

The concept of follicular inflammation with associated intrafollicular mucin dates back to the early 20th century. Kreibich described the case of a 24-year-old man with plaques on the truncal area. The photograph illustrating the clinical and microscopic findings clearly shows the hair follicle to be enveloped by a lymphocytic infiltrate with abundant mucinous change in and adjacent to the follicle.[3] The clinical resemblance to mycosis fungoides (MF) is striking, but there was no clear epidermal involvement with atypical lymphocytes to suggest a diagnosis of MF. Several years later, a similar case was described by Lehner and Szodoray. Once again, the process was reported in a young man, and the course was benign.[4] For several years, Macauley followed a patient who first developed papules located over the eyebrow in association with hair loss. The microscopic picture was that of a primarily follicular-centered infiltrate with abundant intrafollicular mucinosis. After several years, the lesions resolved and hair growth resumed in the involved area. This patient became the index case in the series of seven cases reported by Pinkus as "alopecia mucinosa."[1] Pinkus used this term to emphasize the clinical findings of hair loss and the microscopic changes of follicular mucinosis (FM). He emphasized the clinical picture of slowly evolving, asymptomatic, well-defined plaques. The mucin was reported to first become visible in the outer root sheath area and then the sebaceous gland and was shown to be hyaluronic acid. Eventually this process could result in destruction of the follicle. MF was not mentioned in this report as being part of the pathologic process of alopecia mucinosa. Later the same year, Braun-Falco reported four patients with a similar condition that he described as mucophanerosis follicularis et seboglandularis.[2] The term "phanerosis" implied that the mucin became more visible in this condition, perhaps as a result of degeneration of the follicular structure. Two of these cases had MF associated with the follicular mucin changes. Braun-Falco divided this condition into those cases that were symptomatic of MF (secondary to MF) and those that were primary or idiopathic. Jablonska et al. described another case and used the term "mucinosis follicularis" to describe the microscopic findings.[5] Since these early descriptions, the terms "primary" or "secondary" FM have been used to separate those patients who have no clear evidence for MF from those who do have lymphoma. Emmerson separated the 47 cases in his report into three tiers, those with MF or malignancy, those with persistent disease but no lymphoma, and those with self-limited disease.[6] Coskey and Mehregan described their experience with alopecia mucinosa in 50 patients. They reported a prevalence of MF in approximately 14%. It appeared up to that time that patients younger than 40 years of age and those with lesions limited to the facial area were not as likely to develop MF.[7] Although FM in the strict sense is a histopathologic term, it has been used more often than the term alopecia mucinosa in recent years to describe this process of intrafollicular inflammation with mucin deposition. FM has been used perhaps incorrectly as a synonym for alopecia mucinosa.[8] The precise terminology to best describe this disorder is still a matter of debate.

7.2 CLINICAL

FM occurs in patients of any age, with a male predominance of approximately 2:1. Several clinical patterns are possible. The earliest, most subtle lesion is a single follicular-centered papule (Figure 7.1). Several papules may coalesce into plaques. In hair-bearing areas, there may be partial or complete alopecia. The hair follicles may become more prominent and can be dilated or appear to be plugged. Terminal hair may be replaced by vellus hair. In more severely affected areas, the hair follicle may be completely replaced by a keratinous plug. Typically, the areas of involvement are well-defined and may slowly expand. The skin may be slightly reddish or may appear to be simply swollen and translucent (Figure 7.2). At times, the mucin can be seen grossly in the superficial areas of the skin and can even extrude through the follicular orifice (Figure 7.3). There may be a light, superficial scale, but symptoms are not prominent, as might be expected with eczema. Lichen spinulosa-like lesions, pityriasis-alba-like changes, alopecia areata-like lesions, especially of the scalp, and acneiform or rosacea-like lesions of the face have all been reported (Figures 7.4 and 7.5). The head and neck areas are common sites for initial lesions,

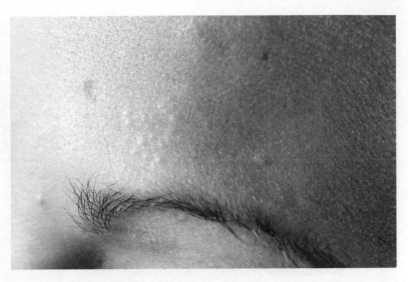

FIGURE 7.1 Cluster of small papules on the forehead shown to represent follicular mucinosis on biopsy.

but the location of initial/primary lesions has not been a reliable marker of association with malignancy.[9,10,11,12,13,14] FM may be seen in children and adolescents (ages 10 to 20 years). Most often, these young patients present with dermatitic-appearing plaques on the head, neck, or extremities. Papular lesions with a strong clinical resemblance to acne of the head and neck have been described (Figures 7.3 and 7.6). FM that begins in childhood can persist for several decades and has occurred in persons with Hodgkin's disease.[15,16,17]

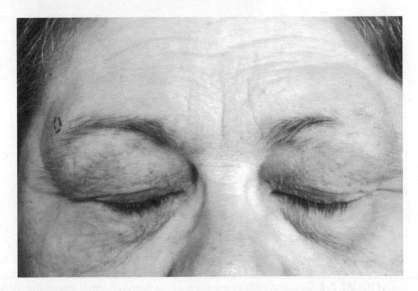

FIGURE 7.2 Edematous plaques of the forehead with partial alopecia of the eyebrows.

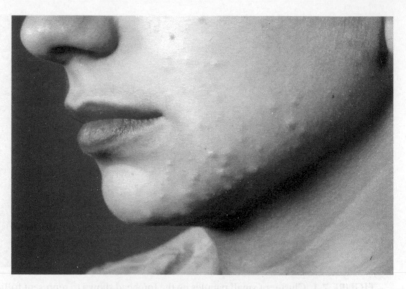

FIGURE 7.3 Discrete and grouped papules containing clear, mucinous material.

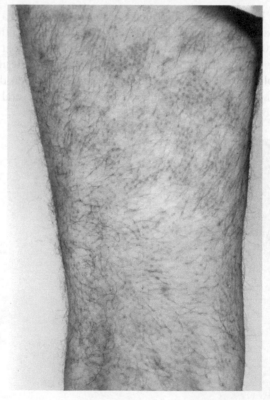

FIGURE 7.4 Grouped follicular lesions of the posterior thigh resembling lichen spinulosus.

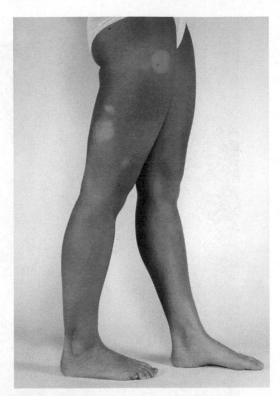

FIGURE 7.5 Hypopigmented annular plaques resembling pityriasis alba or alopecia areata with hypopigmentation.

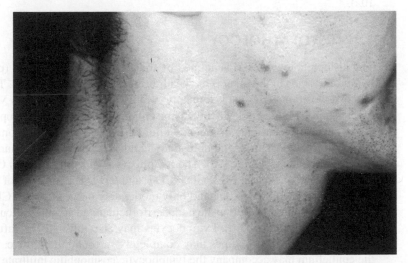

FIGURE 7.6 Papular lesions, alopecia resembling alopecia areata, and dermatitis-like areas on the cheek and neck in follicular mucinosis. (From Wittenberg, G. et al. *J. Am. Acad. Dermatol.* 38, 849, 1998. With permission.)

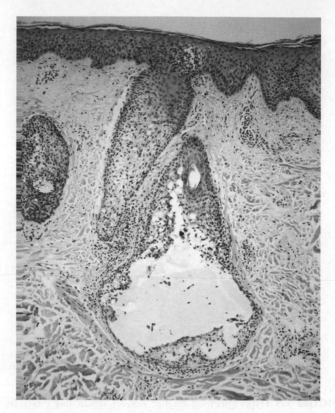

FIGURE 7.7 Follicular mucinosis with abundant intrafollicular mucin deposition (H&E, 10×).

7.3 HISTOPATHOLOGY

The histopathology of FM is defined by the accumulation of mucin (predominantly hyaluronic acid) in the outer root sheath or the sebaceous apparatus. The amount of mucin deposition varies but is typically copious enough to be readily visible without mucin stains (Figure 7.7). Mucin may be emphasized with acid mucopolysaccharide stains such as alcian blue or Hale's colloidal iron. Most lesions contain a mild to moderate folliculocentric lymphohistiocytic infiltrate involving primarily the middle third of the follicle (Figure 7.8). The lymphocytes generally express CD4 and other T-cell markers, including CD3, CD5, CD7, and CD8. The majority of the cells stain predominantly with CD3/CD4 and only moderately or weakly with CD7/CD8 (Figure 7.9). In addition, there may be both perifollicular and an intrafollicular infiltration of eosinophils (Figure 7.10). Lymphocytes may also infiltrate the infundibular portion of the follicle and at times may completely surround the follicle. Spongiosis of the epithelium may accompany the lymphocytic/eosinophilic infiltrate causing some difficulty in separation from dermatitis. Pautrier's collections may be seen in the overlying epidermis in those cases in which the FM is secondary to MF (Figure 7.11). Attempts at separating benign or primary cases of FM from MF based on

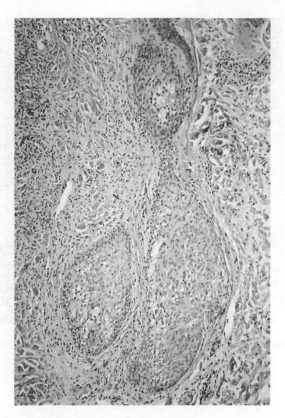

FIGURE 7.8 Follicular mucin with intrafollicular lymphocytic infiltrate and surrounding dermal lymphocytic and eosinophilic infiltrate (H&E, 25×). (From Wittenberg, G. et al. *J. Am. Acad. Dermatol.* 38, 849, 1998. With permission.)

lymphocytic cytologic atypia have generally not been successful. Additional criteria studied have included the amount of follicular mucin, density of eosinophils and density of the lymphocytic infiltrate. No single criterion distinguished MF-associated FM from the primary type. The presence of Pautrier's collections of atypical lymphocytes in the overlying epidermis and/or the infundibulum seen in the same biopsy specimen as FM appears to be the only uniformly accepted histologic criterion for MF. More commonly, several biopsies may be needed to confirm MF in the setting of FM.[6,7,9,10,12]

7.4 MOLECULAR GENETICS

Gene rearrangement studies have demonstrated T-cell clonality (TCR+) in both MF-associated FM and primary FM. Papular or acneiform lesions in young persons have also demonstrated clonality by both fresh-tissue Southern technique as well as by polymerase chain reaction. Clonality does not appear to reliably predict the duration of disease or progression to MF.[9,11–14] The percentage of FM patients with

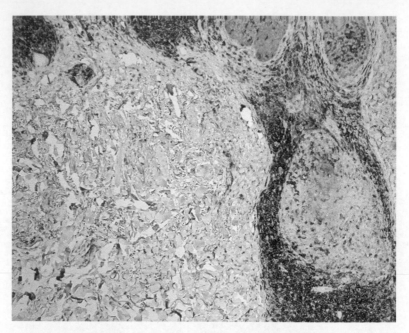

FIGURE 7.9 Pilotropic CD4 lymphocytes in follicular mucinosis (immunoperoxidase, CD4, 25×).

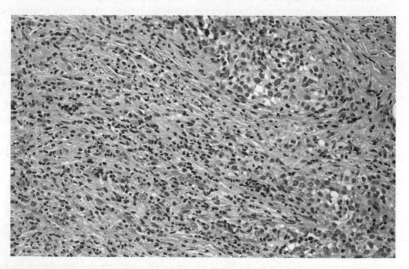

FIGURE 7.10 Higher power view (H&E, 40×) demonstrating numerous eosinophils admixed with lymphocytes in follicular mucinosis.

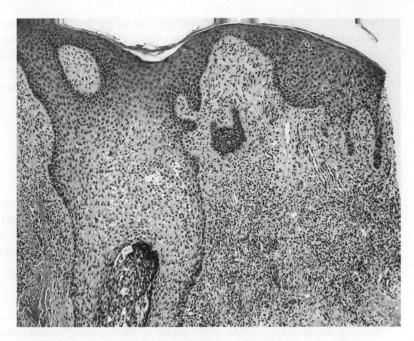

FIGURE 7.11 Mycosis fungoides and follicular mucinosis demonstrating areas of epidermotropism of lymphocytes in addition to pilotropism (H&E, 25×).

inadequate sampling (related to the need to study follicles as opposed to the entire tissue), relative sparsity of lymphocytes in the study sample, and the sensitivity of the test itself.

7.5 DIFFERENTIAL DIAGNOSIS

The diagnosis of FM is based on a combination of characteristic clinical and histopathologic findings. Clinically, alopecia must be present, although in areas such as the forehead this may be difficult to appreciate. Microscopically, the presence of mucin in the follicular apparatus is required for the diagnosis. Rosacea or acneiform eruptions may sometimes closely mimic FM. However, there is often less accumulation of mucin in the follicles of these acneiform eruptions, which typically also show perifollicular plasmacytic or polymorphonuclear cell infiltrates as well as occasional granuloma formation, separating these entities from FM. Various disorders, including eczema, lichen planus, and lupus erythematosus, may at times demonstrate FM as part of the microscopic picture. Follicular or pilotropic MF may resemble FM.[18–27] Pilotropic MF is characterized clinically by grouped follicular papules that may show varying degrees of follicular plugging and, in the fully developed state, replacement of hair with small milia or cysts. The histopathology demonstrates outer root sheath infiltration with atypical lymphocytes, and little to no mucin deposition. Most often, the lymphocytic infiltrate is composed almost entirely of CD4+ cells, and the infundibular area as well as deeper portions of the follicle are involved. Some consider pilotropic MF to be a mucin-poor form of follicular MF and would "lump" these conditions together in the category of follicular MF.[13,24] Eosinophilic pustular folliculitis, or Ofuji's disease, is another diagnostic consideration, as this entity may present with papulopustules in an annular configuration on the face. However, eosinophilic folliculitis is characterized by follicular infiltration of numerous eosinophils, with spongiosis of the follicular epithelium. Furthermore, in eosinophilic folliculitis, mucin deposition is sparse and eosinophils outnumber lymphocytes.[28-30]

7.6   FM AND MALIGNANCY

The association of FM with reticulosis or malignancy has been a subject of interest for the past 75 years. Braun-Falco reported four patients with FM, and two of them had MF.[2] Approximately 15% to 30% of patients with FM reported in case series through the 1990s had or eventually developed MF. Some patients were thought to have primary FM and then eventuated into MF.[32-34] In recent years the reported percentage of patients with FM and MF has increased to over 50%.[12,13] These figures may vary because of referral bias or perhaps because of the flux in the definition of MF. The actual percentage of patients who have MF and FM will depend upon refining the definition of MF in the setting of FM utilizing reproducible criteria and perhaps upon improvements in molecular technologies. FM has also been reported in patients with B-cell lymphoma, chronic lymphocytic leukemia, and Hodgkin's disease.[6,7,9,12,13,15,17] The relationship between FM and B-cell lymphoma is not known.

7.7   TREATMENT

The course of FM is usually chronic and unpredictable. Many treatments have been reported, but most have met with inconsistent results. Therapeutic options, associated with variable success, include potent topical or intralesional corticosteroids, phototherapy with psoralen ultraviolet A (PUVA), combination of low-dose retinoids and PUVA (RePUVA), and PUVA with topical nitrogen mustard.[35] Superficial radiotherapy has been used for decades, but recurrences are likely.[13] Interferon has been reported to be helpful.[36] The literature also contains anecdotes of improvement with dapsone or with acne regimens such as topical retinoids combined with oral tetracyclines.[37-39] Topical bexarotene (Targretin) has recently been reported to be helpful in the treatment of FM and pilotropic MF.[40] MF-associated FM is treated in accordance with protocols used for the appropriate stage of cutaneous T-cell lymphoma.

7.8   SUMMARY AND CONCLUSIONS

In summary, from the historical standpoint FM began as a histopathologic term, but it has since been used to describe what was named alopecia mucinosa by Pinkus. The process of FM is not a degenerative one but is the consequence of a certain type of inflammation involving the epidermal, follicular, and other epithelial structures of the skin. The cause of this disorder is not known, and no infectious origin has been identified as of yet. All patients with primary or idiopathic FM despite the diminutive nature of their lesions are at risk for a T-cell clonal disorder. Patients who were thought to have transformed into MF in the past may have had T-cell clonal disease from the inception of their skin lesions and so may have simply evolved from clonal disease to MF. This disorder overtly challenges our ability to draw a dividing line between those patients who have "primary" FM and those who have MF with the secondary change of FM. Consensus regarding the criteria for the diagnosis of MF in the setting of FM will have to be reached. For now, a combination of clinical, histopathologic, and perhaps molecular criteria are best used to identify those patients at an early state who have MF. When in doubt, it seems best to maintain FM as the primary "provisional" or "working" diagnosis and to follow these patients closely. As concluded by Emmerson, "In view of the entirely benign nature of the condition in the majority of patients, and the spontaneous resolution of lesions in all age groups, it would seem unreasonable to stress the sinister implications of FM, as has been done by some workers."[6]

REFERENCES

1. Pinkus, H. Alopecia mucinosa. *Arch. Dermatol.* 76, 419, 1957.
2. Braun-Falco, O. Mucophanerosis intrafollicularis et seboglandularis. *Dermatologische Wochenschrift* 136, 1289, 1957.
3. Kreibich, C. Mucin bei Hauterkrankung. *Arch. Derm. U. Syph.* 150, 243, 1926.
4. Lehner, E., Szodoray, L. Ein ungewohnlicher, sich durch entzundliches follicularodem auszeichnender hautausschlag. *Derm. Wschr.* 108, 679, 1939.
5. Jablonska, S., Chorzelski, T., and Lanucki, J. Mucinosis follicularis. *Hautarzt.* 10, 27, 1959.
6. Emmerson, R.W. Follicular mucinosis: a study of 47 patients. *Br. J. Dermatol.* 81, 395, 1969.
7. Coskey, R.J. and Mehregan, A.H. Alopecia mucinosa: a follow-up study. *Arch. Dermatol.* 102, 193, 1970.
8. Hempstead, R.W. and Ackerman, A.B. Follicular mucinosis. A reactive pattern in follicular epithelium. *Am. J. Dermatopathol.* 7, 245, 1985.
9. Gibson, L.E. et al. Follicular mucinosis: clinical and histopathologic study. *J. Am. Acad. Dermatol.* 20, 441, 1989.
10. Mehregan, D.A., Gibson, L.E., and Muller, S.A. Follicular mucinosis: Histopathologic review of 33 cases. *Mayo Clin. Proc.* 66, 387, 1991.
11. Wittenberg, G. et al. Follicular mucinosis presenting as an acneiform eruption: report of four cases. *J. Am. Acad. Dermatol.* 38, 849, 1998.
12. Cerroni, L. et al. Follicular mucinosis: A critical reappraisal of clinicopathologic features and association with mycosis fungoides and Sézary syndrome. *Arch. Dermatol.* 138, 182, 2002.
13. van Doorn, R., Scheffer, E., and Willemze, R. Follicular mycosis fungoides, a distinct entity with or without associated follicular mucinosis: a clinicopathologic and follow-up study of 51 patients. *Arch. Dermatol.* 138, 191, 2002.
14. Brown, H.A. et al. Primary follicular mucinosis: long term follow up of patients under 40 years of age with and without clonal T-cell receptor gene rearrangement. *J. Am. Acad. Dermatol.* 47, 856, 2002.

15. Kim, R. and Winkelmann, R.K. Follicular mucinosis (alopecia mucinosa). *Arch. Dermatol.* 85, 490, 1962.
16. Nickoloff, B.J. and Wood C. Benign idiopathic versus mycosis fungoides-associated follicular mucinosis. *Pediatr. Dermatol.* 2, 201, 1985.
17. Gibson, L.E., Muller, S.A., and Peters, M.S. Follicular mucinosis of childhood and adolescence. *Pediatr. Dermatol.* 5, 231, 1988.
18. Wilkinson, J.D., Black, M.M., and Chu, A. Follicular mucinosis associated with mycosis fungoides presenting with gross cystic changes on the face. *Clin. Exp. Dermatol.* 7, 333, 1982.
19. Lacour, J.-P. et al. Follicular mycosis fungoides. A clinical and histologic variant of cutaneous T-cell lymphoma: Report of two cases. *J. Am. Acad. Dermatol.* 29, 330, 1993.
20. Goldenhersh, M.A., Zlotogorski, A., and Rosenmamm, E. Follicular mycosis fungoides. *Am. J. Dermatol.* 16, 52, 1994.
21. Oliviecki, S. and Ashworth, J. Mycosis fungoides with a widespread follicular eruption, comedones and cysts. *Br. J. Dermatol.* 127, 54, 1992.
22. Vergier, B. et al. Pilotropic T cell lymphoma without mucinosis: A variant of mycosis fungoides? *Arch. Dermatol.* 132, 683, 1996.
23. Pereyo, N.G. et al. Follicular mycosis fungoides: a clinicohistopathologic study. *J. Am. Acad. Dermatol.* 36, 563, 1997.
24. Kossard, S. and Rubel, D. Folliculotropic T-cell lymphocytosis (mucin-poor follicular mucinosis). *Australasian J. Dermatol.* 41, 120, 2000.
25. Fraser-Andrews, E., Ashton, R., and Russell-Jones, R. Pilotropic mycosis fungoides presenting with multiple cysts, comedones and alopecia. *Br. J. Dermatol.* 140, 141, 1999.
26. Klemke, C.D. et al. Follicular mycosis fungoides. *Br. J. Dermatol.* 141, 137, 1999.
27. Hodak, E. et al. Follicular cutaneous T-cell lymphoma: a clinicopathological study of nine cases. *Br. J. Dermatol.* 141, 315, 1999.
28. Ofuji, S. et al. Eosinophilic pustular folliculitis. *Acta. Derm. Venereol.* 50, 195, 1970.
29. Buezo, G.F. et al. HIV-associated eosinophilic folliculitis and follicular mucinosis. *Dermatol.* 197, 178, 1998.
30. Lee, J.Y.-Y., Tsai, Y.-M., and Sheu, H.-M. Ofuji's disease with follicular mucinosis and its differential diagnosis from alopecia mucinosa. *J. Cutaneous Pathol.* 30, 307, 2003.
31. Binnick, A.N., Wax, F.D., and Clendenning, W.E. Alopecia mucinosa of the face associated with mycosis fungoides. *Arch. Dermatol.* 114, 791, 1978.
32. Kanno, S. et al. Follicular mucinosis developing into cutaneous lymphoma: report of two cases and review of the literature and 64 cases in Japan. *Acta. Derm. Venereol. (Stockh.)* 64, 86, 1984.
33. Bonta, M.D. et al. Rapidly progressing mycosis fungoides presenting as follicular mucinosis. *J. Am. Acad. Dermatol.* 43, 635, 2000.
34. Leman, J.A. and Mackie, R.M. A case of follicular mucinosis progressing to mycosis fungoides (poster). *Clin. Exp. Dermatol.* 27, 225, 2002.
35. Kenicer, K.J.A. and Lakshmipathi, T. Follicular mucinosis treated with PUVA. *Br. J. Dermatol.* 107, 48, 1982.
36. Meissner, K. et al. Successful treatment of primary progressive follicular mucinosis with interferons. *J. Am. Acad. Dermatol.* 24, 848, 1991.
37. Kubba, R.K. and Stewart, T.W. Follicular mucinosis responding to dapsone. *Br. J. Dermatol.* 91, 217, 1974.

38. Rustin, M.H., Bunker, C.B., and Levene, G.M. Follicular mucinosis presenting as acute dermatitis and response to dapsone. *Clin. Exp. Dermatol.* 14, 382, 1989.
39. Yotsumoto, S., Uchimiya, H., and Kanzaki, T. A case of follicular mucinosis treated successfully with minocycline. *Br. J. Dermatol.* 142, 841, 2000.
40. Hanson, M., Hill, A., and Duvic, M. Bexarotene reverses alopecia in cutaneous T-cell lymphoma. *Br. J. Dermatol.* 149, 193, 2003.

8 Immunohistochemistry and Molecular Biologic Techniques for Diagnosis, Staging, and Monitoring of Cutaneous T-Cell Lymphoma

H.L. Greenberg and Gary S. Wood

CONTENTS

8.1 NOMENCLATURE

Immunohistochemistry and molecular biological techniques are becoming ever more powerful and important tools for distinguishing different types of cutaneous T-cell lymphoma (CTCL). Currently, these techniques are in the early phases of use for staging and monitoring CTCL. We believe that in the future, immunohistochemistry and molecular biological techniques will be utilized increasingly for these purposes as well as for diagnosis. Before we detail the techniques and their implications, we review the nomenclature involved.

CTCL encompasses primary and secondary skin involvement by different forms of T-cell lymphomas; however, this term is used mainly in reference to mycosis fungoides (MF) and its leukemic variant, Sezary syndrome.[1-4] Two types of characterizations are used: immunophenotypic and immunogenotypic. Lymphoid antigen expression is the basis for immunophenotyping — monoclonal antibodies are used in order to identify the immunophenotype, typically using the cluster of differentiation (CD) antigen designations. T-cell receptor (TCR) gene rearrangements and select chromosomal translocations are the basis for immunogenotyping. Dominant T-cell clones are usually identified with polymerase chain reaction (PCR)-based gene amplification techniques.

8.2 IMMUNOPHENOTYPING

Different T-cell markers are used in order to identify T-cell subsets. By using the various CD markers, investigators are able to recognize T-cell origin. Typically, CTCL involves postthymic, memory, helper T cells belonging to the skin-associated lymphoid tissue (SALT).[4] SALT T cells traffic throughout the skin, peripheral lymphoid tissue, blood vessels, and lymphatics. Cutaneous lymphocyte antigen (CLA) expression identifies T cells involved in the SALT. T-cell CLA and endothelial cell E-selectin serve a receptor-ligand function in the dermal microvasculature, allowing T cells to traffic throughout the skin. By identifying CD markers on the T cells, investigators are able to determine the nature of these T cells. Postthymic T cells are notable for their lack of TdT, CD1a, and CD4/CD8 co-expression. Well-differentiated T cells demonstrate CD2, CD3, and CD5 expression. Memory T cells express CD45RO, while helper T cells express CD4. The memory effector subset of helper T cells lacks CD62L, whereas the memory recall subset does not. Other less well-defined markers may prove useful for identifying tumor cells in the future. Some of these markers reported to be deficient in CTCL include CD26 and CD49d, whereas positive markers include CD60.[5,6]

Distinguishing features of CTCL typically include variations on the T-cell immunophenotypic characteristics discussed above. Whereas well-differentiated T cells are notable for CD2, CD3, and CD5 expression, a small proportion of CTCL cells lack one or more of these markers. CD3 is often expressed less intensely in CTCL than the other two markers, giving rise to the "CD3-dim" phenotype.

Typically, CTCL cells lack the CD7 marker. In fact, having less than 30% of T cells CD7 positive is a moderately sensitive and specific marker for CTCL.[7,8] Having an even lower percentage (less than 10%) of CD7-positive T cells is, in our experience, more specific but also less sensitive for CTCL.[7] Reduced CD7 is typical of CTCL, as noted in previous studies,[7,9] and can also be seen to varying extents in chronic inflammatory cutaneous T-cell infiltrates. This association between chronic inflammation and CTCL suggests that similar T-cell subsets may be involved in both of these processes. Another feature shared by some normal, inflammatory, and CTCL T cells is CD62L (L-selectin) negativity.[7,10]

More T-cell markers are available for frozen sections or flow cytometry samples than markers for paraffin sections, resulting in frozen sections and flow cytometry's being the preferred methods of antigen identification. However, T-cell identification in paraffin sections is improving because of an increasing number of anti T-cell antibodies that work well in paraffin sections. Commercially available antibodies usable in formalin-fixed, paraffin-embedded tissue sections include pan-T-cell markers, major T-cell subset markers, and even CD7.[11] Immunohistology is preferred over flow cytometry for the diagnostic evaluation of skin specimens because of architectural preservation. Differential diagnosis is aided by the retention of architectural detail and is less likely to result in sampling artifact seen during creation of cell suspensions from solid tissues.

8.3 IMMUNOGENOTYPING

Lymphomas arise genetically from a single clone. It has been determined that TCR gene rearrangement studies can reliably assess clonality.[12–16]

TCR gene rearrangement involves the internal reorganization of alpha, beta, gamma, and delta TCR genes during T-cell differentiation. Gamma/delta rearrangement, followed by alpha/beta rearrangement, occurs as part of the maturing process in CTCL cells and about 95% of mature peripheral T cells. The TCR-delta gene is embedded within the TCR-alpha gene and is, as a result, lost during alpha gene rearrangement. Although it is no longer expressed, the TCR-gamma gene, which has also undergone rearrangement, is retained within alpha/beta-expressing T cells including CTCL cells. Because of its retention, TCR-gamma gene rearrangements can be analyzed in CTCL. In fact, the TCR gamma gene is less complex than the alpha or beta genes, resulting in technically easier molecular biologic assays targeting this gene.[14]

Many different assays have been developed to determine the clonality of TCR gene rearrangements.[13] We discuss three assays here: Southern blot analysis (SBA), PCR-based amplification of TCR-gamma gene rearrangements followed by ribonuclease protection analysis (PCR/RPA), and our preferred method, PCR-based amplification of TCR-gamma genes followed by denaturing gradient gel electrophoresis (PCR/DGGE). Measured as a percentage of clonal DNA, the clonal detection threshold of the aforementioned assays is each different and is used to determine monoclonality and polyclonality as a positive and negative result, respectively.

The SBA technique was the first one used for the analysis of CTCL TCR gene rearrangement; however, the PCR-based techniques are more sensitive. Under the best circumstances, SBA has a clonality detection threshold of approximately 5%, but it can be as poor as 10% to 20%; this low sensitivity will not detect clonality in early (patch-stage) CTCL.[14] PCR/RPA has a highly sensitive clonal detection threshold approximating 1/100,000 cells.[15] Because of this highly sensitive threshold, the PCR/RPA assay can detect clonal CTCL cells in samples of allergic contact dermatitis and clinicopathologically normal lymphoid tissues obtained from CTCL patients.[12] Clinical relevancy for clonal detection occurs at a sensitivity near 1%. PCR/DGGE has a sensitivity threshold near 1%, and in up to 90% of CTCL cases, it will demonstrate dominant clonality.[14,16] The reasons for false negatives include failure of PCR primers to detect all possible gene rearrangements, tumor cell density below the detection threshold, and the absence or deletion of TCR-gamma gene rearrangements.

One of the pitfalls in testing for clonality is ensuring that the results are interpreted in the proper clinical and histopathologic context. A positive result (dominant clonality) may occur, but on histopathologic examination, there may be chronic dermatitis instead of CTCL. In such cases, the term "clonal dermatitis" is used.[14] Patients with clonal dermatitis have a 20% risk of developing overt CTCL within 5 years.[17] Clonal precursors to overt lymphoma have been observed in entities other than clonal dermatitis including lymphoid hyperplasia, lymphomatoid papulosis, monoclonal gammopathy of uncertain significance, and angioimmunoblastic lymphadenopathy with dysproteinemia.[14]

8.4 CTCL DIAGNOSTIC CRITERIA

In an effort to better categorize early (patch/thin plaque) MF, an integration of the immunophenotypic and immunogenotypic findings, in addition to the current CTCL criteria, is being formulated. The International Society for Cutaneous Lymphomas (ISCL) is currently spearheading this early MF categorization effort, although it is not yet complete. A precursor algorithm has been developed that could serve as a working model that will be modified when improved criteria from future studies prove the need (see Table 8.1). Erythrodermic and Sezary syndrome CTCL criteria have been modified recently based upon criteria developed and published elsewhere by the ISCL (Table 8.2).[10] In erythrodermic CTCL, the hematologic findings include disease with or without leukemia, percentage of Sezary cells, T-cell clonality or karyotypic abnormality, and specific CD marker T-cell deficiencies.[10]

8.5 STAGING OF CTCL

The current tumor-node-metastasis (TNM) staging system for CTCL is based on a combination of two sets of clinicopathologic data: first, the type and extent of skin involvement and, second, the presence or absence of nodal and visceral disease (Table 8.3).[18] This staging system has been used for prognostication in numerous studies (similar to those outlined in Table 8.1).[4] Unfortunately, using the same criteria in the viscera, lymph nodes, and skin lesions leads to some diagnostic problems. Attempts at using immunophenotypic and immunogenotypic characteristics as ancillary staging criteria may facilitate an enhanced sensitivity and/or specificity beyond the histopathologic criteria.[19-23] Abnormal T-cell antigen expression patterns and dominant clonality are the criteria used for staging CTCL in such cases.[4] It has been suggested by some preliminary studies that using such ancillary staging methods provides additional prognostic information when compared to obtaining histopathologic findings alone.[20,21]

As previously discussed, clonality assays vary in terms of their sensitivity; establishing a test that is appropriately sensitive for staging is difficult. The SBA

TABLE 8.1
Early Mycosis Fungoides Diagnostic Algorithm for Patients with Clinically Suspicious Skin Lesions[a]

Diagnosis	T-Cell Receptor Gene Rearrangement	Immunohistochemistry	Histopathology
Mycosis fungoides	+/–	+/–	Mycosis fungoides
Mycosis fungoides	+	+/–	Possible mycosis fungoides
Mycosis fungoides	–	+	Possible mycosis fungoides
LPP[b]	–	–	Possible mycosis fungoides
LPP	–	+/–	Dermatitis
Clonal dermatitis[c]	+	+/–	Dermatitis

Note: T-cell receptor gene rearrangement: + (dominant clonal pattern), – (polyclonal pattern); Immunohistochemistry: + (less than 50% CD2+, CD3+, and/or CD5+; less than 10% CD7+; epidermal/dermal discordance for CD2, CD3, CD5, and/or CD7), – (any other results using these markers).

[a] Discrete, erythematous, variably scaly patches and thin plaques that may be poikilodermatous, of variable size and shape, and/or favor sun-protected skin when limited in distribution.

[b] Includes pseudo-mycosis-fungoides drug eruptions.

[c] Approximately 20% progress to mycosis fungoides over 5 years.

Source: Adapted from Wood, G. S. and Greenberg, H. L. *Dermatol. Ther.* 16, 269, 2003.

TABLE 8.2
Subtypes of Erythrodermic Cutaneous T-Cell Lymphoma

Erythrodermic Subset	Prior Mycosis Fungoides	Hematologic Findings	TNBM B Status	TNBM Stage[a]
Sezary syndrome	Rare	Leukemia	B2	IVA
Erythrodermic mycosis fungoides	Yes	Minimal or absent	B0-1	III[b]
Erythrodermic cutaneous T-cell lymphoma, other	No	Minimal or absent	B0-1	III[b]

Note: B2 criteria include any of the following peripheral blood findings: Sezary cells $\geq 1,000/mm^3$, CD4/CD8 ≥ 10 due to increased T cells; dominant T-cell clone by gene rearrangement or karyotyping; T-cell deficiency of CD2, CD3, CD4, or CD5; an additional tentative criterion is T-cell deficiency of CD7 or an expanded CD4+ CD7– subset $\geq 40\%$. B1 criteria include not meeting B2 criteria, but Sezary cells $\geq 5\%$ lymphocytes plus dominant T-cell clonality. If relying only on Sezary cell counts, then $\geq 20\%$ lymphocytes is required. B0 criteria include any situation other than B1 or B2.

[a] All are T4. Regardless of B status, N2–3 makes the stage IVA, and M1 makes the stage IVB.

[b] IIIA versus IIIB depends on whether N status is 0 or 1, respectively.

Source: Adapted from Bernengo, M.G. et al. *Br. J. Dermatol.* 144, 125, 2001.

TABLE 8.3
Mycosis Fungoides Staging System Tumor-Node-Metastasis (TNM)
Classification Numbers

Stage	Tumor	Node	Metastases
IA	1–Patch/plaque 10%	0–Normal nodes	0–None
IB	2–Patch/plaque > 10%	0–Normal nodes	0–None
IIA	1–2–Patch/plaque — Any	1–Enlarged nodes, mycosis fungoides negative	0–None
IIB	3–Skin tumor(s)	0–1–Normal or enlarged nodes, mycosis fungoides negative	0–None
IIIA	4–Erythroderma	0–Normal nodes	0–None
IIIB	4–Erythroderma	1–Enlarged nodes, mycosis fungoides negative	0–None
IVA	1–4–Any of the above	2–3–Normal-enlarged nodes, mycosis fungoides positive	0–None
IVB	1–4–Any of the above	0–3–Any of the above	1–Viscera involved

Source: Adapted from Tracey, L. et al. *Blood* 102, 1042, 2003.

technique is not sensitive enough, whereas certain PCR techniques are too sensitive. The PCR/RPA assay is too sensitive, in that this assay has shown involvement in microscopically normal lymph nodes, blood, and bone marrow.[15] The PCR/RPA technique was positive in patients who rarely develop clinical involvement of these tissues and have a normal life expectancy because of their early stage IA -limited patch-type CTCL.[15] In cases in which there is no difference in life expectancy or clinical course, having such a sensitive assay is not clinically useful for staging or monitoring disease activity.

Incidental clonal T-cell expansion of uncertain significance (TEXUS) occurs in the peripheral blood of a minority of older individuals and is important to consider in patients at risk for hematologic CTCL involvement.[24,25] CTCL is a CD4-positive disease, whereas TEXUS typically involves CD8-positive T-cell expansion. However, there have also been clonal CD4-positive expansions in patients with miscellaneous hematologic disease unrelated to CTCL. Clonal gene rearrangement matching that in lesional skin must be shown in other tissues such as lymph nodes in order to be classified as CTCL.[23] The ability to match band patterns in different tissues is one of the benefits of the PCR/DGGE assay.[14] Both nucleotide sequence and size are utilized when the urea-formamide gradient within the DGGE gel separates PCR products. Because of this combination of size and nucleotide sequence, the PCR/DGGE technique is superior to other size-based types of electrophoresis for detecting matching clonal bands among multiple samples from the same patient.

8.6 MONITORING CTCL-DISEASE ACTIVITY

It is becoming clear that solely relying upon clinical assessment is inadequate for identifying residual CTCL. Invisible CTCL may be seen on histopathologic examination of the clinically uninvolved skin of patients with either active CTCL or occult residual disease.[26] Because there are relapses of CTCL in patients who had been clinically disease free, it is common practice to continue therapy for months or years after achieving clinical remission. Both immunophenotypic and immunogenotypic assays are able to detect relapse and monitor therapy response.[13] In addition, these techniques may be used to define remission more accurately in the future.[13]

8.7 THE FUTURE

Validation of the current system of diagnosing and staging CTCL is ongoing. We have yet to fully utilize the powerful molecular techniques at our disposal for the detection of CTCL. We are also moving toward an age of quantitative instead of qualitative molecular biologic techniques. In the future, there will be more of an emphasis placed on clinically relevant quantitative thresholds for disease detection. Until recently, we were limited in our analysis by detecting only single genes. A new age of technology has now emerged in terms of identifying gene expression. Ideally, through the use of gene chips and microarrays, we will be able to detect coordinated gene expression.

Using complementary DNA (cDNA) arrays, it is possible to identify both gene over- and underexpression. Arrays are arrangements of cDNA oligonucleotides in an orderly fashion. The naming of arrays is based upon sample spot size. The micro versus macro designation is based on a spot size of less than 200 versus greater than 300 microns in diameter, respectively.[27,28] Real-time reverse transcriptase PCR (RT/PCR) is a quantitative measure of gene expression that can be used to verify DNA microarrays.[29] This technology is currently in the experimental stage, but it may some day be another tool in the staging and prognostication of CTCL. A study by Tracey et al. identified 27 genes through cDNA microarry, which correlated with a clinicopathologic diagnosis of MF.[30] In the same article, they were also able to separate inflammatory dermatoses and MF with 97% accuracy using only 6 genes.[30] In a different study by Kari et al. the authors identified 10 genes, with cDNA arrays that were associated with shorter survival times in patients with Sezary syndrome.[31] Kari et al. also noted that Th2-specific genes were overexpressed, while CD26, Stat-4, and IL-1 receptors were all underexpressed.[31]

One of the issues involved in the preparation of samples is determining which sample areas house the affected genes. In order to identify genes involved in CTCL, Storz et al. identified and cultured lymphocytes from MF tumors.[32] Through cDNA microarray techniques they discovered constitutive expression of CD40 and CD40L in neoplastic but not normal lymphocytes.[32] While some authors advocate targeted laser capture microdissection of involved cells,[29] other authors use whole skin biopsies, subtracting the values found in normal skin as a type of background noise.[30] In a recent article by Dereure et al. the authors used hand microdissection with a 30-gauge needle under 40 times magnification in order to localize the areas to be tested.[33] Dereure et al. noted that in using their hand microdissection technique, previously missed cases of MF were reclassified, increasing the percentage of clonal MF cases from 55% to 83% when microdissected DNA was used instead of the sample as a whole.[33] "Micromolecular" analysis of specimens through the use of real-time PCR and laser capture microdissection will be helpful in identifying enriched cell populations that are free from background contamination.

Some of the problems inherent in this technology include identifying what is normal, what is involved tissue, and what is the appropriate standard. King et al. noted that cDNA microarrays demonstrate gene expression; however, this may not be physiologically relevant.[29] Also, it is important to note that proteins and posttranslational modifications are not identified in this process. Identifying the genes "at risk" is possible with all of the aforementioned techniques. As the technology develops, we will increase our collective data set and gain a greater understanding of the pathogenesis and behavior of CTCL. We will become better able to determine the natural course of disease and predict which therapies will be most effective. Ultimately, our ability to diagnose, monitor, and characterize CTCL will improve significantly.

ACKNOWLEDGMENTS

This research was supported by National Institutes of Health Grants AR02136 and CA89442 and Merit Review funding from the Department of Veterans Affairs.

REFERENCES

1. Harris, N.L. et al. A revised European–American classification of lymphoid neoplasms: a proposal from the International Lymphoma Study Group. *Blood* 84, 1361, 1994.
2. Willemze, R. et al. EORTC classification for primary cutaneous lymphomas: a proposal from the Cutaneous Lymphoma Study Group of the European Organization for Research and Treatment of Cancer. *Blood* 90, 354, 1997.
3. Jaffe, E. *WHO Classification of Tumors: Pathology and Genetics of Tumors of Hematopoietic and Lymphoid Tissues*, IARC Press, Lyon, 2001.
4. Wood, G.S. The benign and malignant cutaneous lymphoproliferative disorders including mycosis fungoides, in *Neoplastic Hematopathology*, 2nd ed., Knowles, D.M., Ed., Williams & Wilkins, Baltimore, 2001, p. 1183.
5. Bernengo, M.G. et al. The relevance of the CD4+ CD26– subset in the identification of circulating Sezary cells. *Br. J. Dermatol.* 144, 125, 2001.
6. Scala, E. et al. T cell receptor-Vbeta analysis identifies a dominant CD60+ CD26– CD49d– T cell clone in the peripheral blood of Sezary syndrome patients. *J. Invest. Dermatol.* 119, 193, 2002.
7. Wood, G.S. et al. Leu-8 and Leu-9 antigen phenotypes: immunologic criteria for the distinction of mycosis fungoides from cutaneous inflammation. *J. Am. Acad. Dermatol.* 14, 1006, 1986.
8. Bergman, R. et al. Immunophenotyping and T-cell receptor gamma gene rearrangement analysis as an adjunct to the histopathologic diagnosis of mycosis fungoides. *J. Am. Acad. Dermatol.* 39, 554, 1998.
9. Rappl, G. et al. CD4(+) CD7(–) T cells compose the dominant T-cell clone in the peripheral blood of patients with Sezary syndrome. *J. Am. Acad. Dermatol.* 44, 456, 2001.

10. Vonderheid, E.C. et al. Update on erythrodermic cutaneous T-cell lymphoma: report of the International Society for Cutaneous Lymphomas. *J. Am. Acad. Dermatol.* 46, 95, 2002.

11. Ormsby, A. et al. Evaluation of a new paraffin-reactive CD7 T-cell deletion marker and a polymerase chain reaction-based T-cell receptor gene rearrangement assay: implications for diagnosis of mycosis fungoides in community clinical practice. *J. Am. Acad. Dermatol.* 43, 405, 2001.

12. Veelken, H., Sklar J.L., and Wood, G.S. Detection of low-level tumor cells in allergic contact dermatitis induced by mechlorethamine in patients with mycosis fungoides. *J. Invest. Dermatol.* 106, 685, 1996.

13. Wood, G.S. et al. Molecular biology techniques for the diagnosis of cutaneous T-cell lymphoma. *Dermatol. Clin.* 12, 231, 1994.

14. Wood, G.S. et al. Detection of clonal T-cell receptor gene rearrangements in early mycosis fungoides/Sézary syndrome by polymerase chain reaction and denaturing gradient gel electrophoresis (PCR/DGGE). *J. Invest. Dermatol.* 103, 34, 1994.

15. Veelken, H., Wood, G.S., and Sklar, J. Molecular staging of cutaneous T-cell lymphoma: evidence for systemic involvement in early disease. *J. Invest. Dermatol.,* 104, 889, 1995.

16. Wood, G.S. and Uluer, A.Z. Polymerase chain reaction/denaturing gradient gel electrophoresis (PCR/DGGE): Sensitivity, band pattern analysis and methodologic optimization. *Am. J. Dermatopathol.* 21, 547, 1999.

17. Siddiqui, J. et al. Clonal dermatitis: A potential precursor of CTCL with varied clinical manifestations. *J. Invest. Dermatol.* 108, 584, 1997.

18. Bunn, P.A. and Lamberg, S.I. Report of the committee on staging and classification of cutaneous T-cell lymphomas. *Cancer Treat. Rep.* 63, 725, 1979.

19. Weiss, L., Wood G.S., and Warnke, R.A. Immunophenotypic differences between dermatopathic lymphadenopathy and lymph node involvement in mycosis fungoides. *Am. J. Pathol.* 120, 179, 1985.

20. Kern, D.E. et al. Analysis of T-cell receptor gene rearrangement in lymph nodes of patients with mycosis fungoides: prognostic implications. *Arch. Dermatol.* 134, 158, 1998.

21. Fraser-Andrews, E.A. et al. Detection of a peripheral blood T cell clone is an independent prognostic marker in mycosis fungoides. *J. Invest. Dermatol.* 114, 117, 2000.

22. Muche, J.M. et al. Peripheral blood T cell clonality in mycosis fungoides — an independent prognostic marker? *J. Invest. Dermatol.* 115, 504, 2000.

23. Delfau-Larue, M.H. et al. Prognostic significance of a polymerase chain reaction-detectable dominant T-lymphocyte clone in cutaneous lesions of patients with mycosis fungoides. *Blood* 92, 3376, 1998.

24. Posnett, D.N. et al. Clonal populations of T cells in normal elderly humans: the T cell equivalent to "benign monoclonal gammapathy." *J. Exp. Med.* 179, 609, 1994.

25. Moss, P. et al. Clonal populations of CD4+ and CD8+ T cells in patients with multiple myeloma and paraproteinemia. *Blood* 87, 3297, 1996.

26. Pujol, R.M. et al. Invisible mycosis fungoides: a diagnostic challenge. *J. Am. Acad. Dermatol.* 47 (Suppl. 2), S168, 2002.

27. Shi, L. DNA microarray (genome chip): Monitoring the genome on a chip. http://www.gene-chips.com, 1998–2002.

28. http://www.affymetrix.com.

29. King, H.C. and Sinha, A.A. Gene expression profile analysis by DNA microarrays: Promise and pitfalls. *JAMA* 286, 2280, 2001.

30. Tracey, L. et al. Mycosis fungoides shows concurrent deregulation of multiple genes involved in the TNF signaling pathway: an expression profile study. *Blood* 102, 1042, 2003.
31. Kari, L. et al. Classification and prediction of survival in patients with the leukemic phase of cutaneous T cell lymphoma. *J. Exp. Med.* 197, 1477, 2003.
32. Storz, M. et al. Coexpression of CD40 and CD40 ligand in cutaneous T-cell lymphoma (mycosis mungoides). *Cancer Res.* 61, 452, 2001.
33. Dereure, O. et al. Improved sensitivity of T-cell clonality. Detection in mycosis fungoides by hand microdissection and heteroduplex analysis. *Arch. Dermatol.* 139, 1571, 2003.
34. Wood, G.S. and Greenberg, H.L. Diagnosis, staging, and monitoring of cutaneous T-cell lymphoma. *Dermatol. Ther.* 16, 269, 2003.

9 Molecular Abnormalities

Sean Whittaker

CONTENTS

9.1 INTRODUCTION

The underlying molecular pathogenesis of cutaneous T-cell lymphoma (CTCL) remains elusive, but considerable progress has been made during the past decade with the application of novel molecular techniques. Malignancies are characterized by a series of acquired genetic or epigenetic abnormalities affecting specific genes that control critical cellular functions such as apoptosis, proliferation, and differentiation as well as genome integrity. Such genes can be dysregulated through a combination of mechanisms including mutation, heterozygous or homozygous deletion, and gene amplification. Dysregulation may also occur via fusion of a gene with a powerful promotor such as the IgH gene in the t(9;14) of Burkitt's lymphoma or the creation of a novel fusion gene as a consequence of a chromosomal translocation such as the NPM-ALK fusion gene characteristic of the t(2;5) translocation found in systemic CD30+ anaplastic large cell lymphoma.[1] Such chromosomal translocations are often tumor specific and may represent either a fundamental pathogenetic abnormality or underlying genomic instability that contributes to the cumulative rate of mutations.[2] Importantly, these disease-specific cytogenetic abnormalities are now the focus for the development of tumor-specific therapy, with very encouraging results, as seen in chronic myeloid leukemia with tyrosine kinase inhibitors.[3] Epigenetic abnormalities can also lead to dysregulation of genes through different mechanisms, including hypermethylation of CpG-rich sites within promotor sequences of genes producing transcriptional silencing, generalized hypomethylation of DNA, which may cause aberrant expression of specific genes, and deacetylation of histone proteins, affecting chromatin structure and, consequently, gene transcription. Such abnormalities are attractive therapeutic targets, and there is now considerable interest in the development of phase I/II trials assessing novel therapies that have been shown to reverse these epigenetic changes in tumor cells.

The underlying molecular pathogenetic abnormalities in B-cell non-Hodgkin's lymphoma (NHL) have been shown to often involve genes controlling the proliferation and differentiation of normal B cells. CTCL is one of the most common T-cell malignancies, and it is highly likely that the critical pathogenetic changes involve defects of normal T-cell development. Both mycosis fungoides (MF) and Sezary syndrome share a similar pattern of molecular abnormalities, suggesting that they represent a spectrum of the same disease in contrast to primary cutaneous CD30+ anaplastic large cell lymphoma, which has a distinct pattern.[4,5] However, at present no distinctive molecular features for the different clinical variants of MF have been identified. In MF and Sezary syndrome, there is a high rate of genomic instability as indicated by the presence of both chromosomal and microsatellite instability.[6,7,8] Although no disease-specific translocations have been identified, there is a consistent pattern of chromosomal deletion often associated with unbalanced translocations, suggesting that there is a selection pressure for tumor cells with specific cytogenetic deletions, but the precise genes dysregulated by such defects have yet to be identified. In both MF and Sezary syndrome, there appears to be a preference for abnormalities of genes controlling apoptosis and transcription factors involved specifically in both early and late T-cell activation, which in turn might contribute to defects of activation-induced cell death. This pattern of molecular changes confers a survival advantage for tumor cells, but the disease stage at which these abnormalities occur remains unclear.

9.2 GENOMIC INSTABILITY

Studies in MF and Sezary syndrome have been hindered by an inability to create long-term cultures of tumor cells and an inability to study cytogenetic abnormalities in early stage disease from skin biopsies with relatively low proportions of malignant cells. However, previous G-banded karyotypic studies of peripheral blood tumor metaphases in Sezary syndrome have revealed numerous random and nonrandom structural and numerical abnormalities but no disease-specific balanced translocations.[6] This has been assumed to reflect gross chromosomal instability associated with end-stage malignancy and is a poor prognostic feature, although similar cytogenetic abnormalities have also been detected in metaphases derived from peripheral blood lymphocytes of patients with early stage disease.[9] The complex karyotypic abnormalities detected with G-banding in Sezary syndrome can be resolved partly with multicolor fluorescent in-situ hybridization (M-FISH) analysis, which involves labeling whole chromosomes with fluorescent paints, allowing clarification of complex translocations. M-FISH analysis in Sezary syndrome has revealed frequent involvement of chromosomes 1p, 10q, and 17 in complex unbalanced translocations often associated with deletions[6] (Figure 9.1). Two recurrent but unbalanced translocations — namely, a der(1)t(1;10)(p2;q2) and der(14)t(14;15)(q;q) — have been identified, but it has yet to be established if these translocations have an identical breakpoint to suggest the involvement of a gene or putative fusion gene of funda-

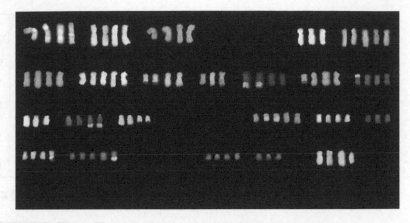

FIGURE 9.1 Multicolor fluorescent in situ hybridization analysis of peripheral blood metaphases from a Sezary syndrome patient showing an aneuploid karyotype with complex unbalanced translocations.

mental pathogenetic importance.[6] Indeed this would be unlikely in view of the deletions associated with both these recurrent translocations.

In primary cutaneous CD30+ large cell anaplastic lymphomas, studies have not identified the NPM-ALK fusion gene characteristic of the t(2;5) translocation present in systemic CD30+ large cell anaplastic lymphoma, consistent with clinical data indicating a different prognosis and distinct pathogenesis.[10]

Comparative genomic hybridization (CGH) techniques provide a means to study gross chromosomal abnormalities in tumor DNA samples using fluorescent DNA labeling and competitive hybridization of tumor and control DNA to high-quality normal metaphases (Figure 9.2).[11] In CTCL several studies have reported a consistent pattern of chromosomal gains and losses that is the same in both MF and Sezary syndrome, suggesting that both disorders represent a spectrum of disease with a similar pathogenesis.[4,12] Chromosomal abnormalities occur in more than 70% of cases and consist of 1p, 10q, 13q, 17p, and 19 losses and frequent gains involving chromosomes 4 and 17q. The loss of 17p and gain of 17q reflects the frequent presence of isochromosome 17 detected with conventional cytogenetics. In contrast, in primary cutaneous CD30+ large cell anaplastic lymphomas (LCALs), CGH studies have shown a different pattern to that found in MF and Sezary syndrome with chromosomal gains and losses in 46% of cases and frequent gains involving 1p and 5.[5]

CGH techniques cannot detect translocations and have a limited ability to resolve small deletions or amplifications. A complementary and widely used approach to defining small regions of deletion is the detection of loss of heterozygosity by polymerase chain reaction (PCR) analysis of a series of highly polymorphic microsatellites in the chromosomal region of interest. In MF, extensive allelotyping studies (Figure 9.3) have identified regions of deletion on 1p, 10q, and 17p, and more detailed analysis has defined two minimal regions of deletion at 10q24 and several different regions on 1p.[4,7,13] In some of these patients, homozygous deletion of the

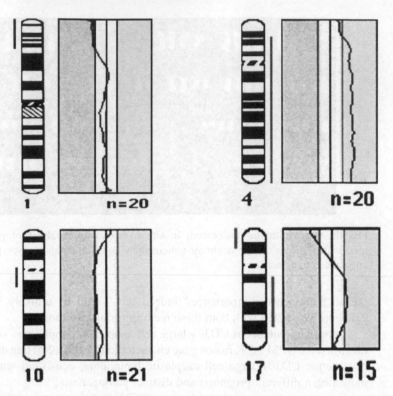

FIGURE 9.2 Comparative genomic hybridization profile illustrating results in a patient with Sezary syndrome showing losses on 1p, 10q, and 17p with gains on 4 and 17q. Results are based on assessment of varying numbers of metaphases (15–21) for each tumor DNA sample compared to control DNA.

PTEN tumor suppressor gene at 10q23 was identified, but further resolution of these regions of deletion and studies of candidate genes are now required.[7] Microsatellite analysis in primary cutaneous CD30+ LCAL has detected deletions at 9p21, suggesting that the p15/16 genes are inactivated.[14]

This approach has also provided evidence of microsatellite instability (MSI) in CTCL (Figure 9.3); Microsatellites, as either mono-, di-, tri- or tetranucleotides, are dispersed throughout the genome and are inherently unstable. A mismatch repair enzyme system is responsible for correcting errors occurring in microsatellite sequences during DNA replication. In hereditary nonpolyposis colorectal cancer (HNPCC) kindreds, one or other of these mismatch repair enzymes (MLH1 or MSH2) is defective, usually because of germline mutations.[15] This contributes to a general level of genomic (nucleotide) instability and causes a mutator phenotype. This mismatch repair enzyme system can be dysregulated in sporadic malignancies and may then prevent the repair of spontaneous mutations, thereby contributing to a higher inherent rate of mutations in the malignant cell. In both MF and Sezary syndrome, MSI has been detected in 24% of tumors,[7,8] suggesting that there is a significant level of nucleotide instability in CTCL as well as a high degree of

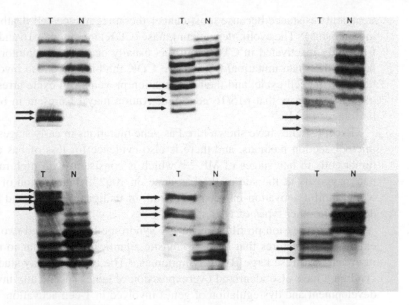

FIGURE 9.3 Autoradiographs showing examples of microsatellite instability (arrows indicating additional bands) detected in tumor DNA samples (T) from patients with mycosis fungoides compared to normal control DNA samples (N) for each patient after amplification with different microsatellite primers.

chromosomal instability indicated by previous cytogenetic studies. Microsatellite instability in CTCL appears to be due to hypermethylation of the MLHI promoter producing transcriptional silencing, rather than inactivating mutations of the gene.[8]

In summary, the consistent pattern of chromosomal abnormalities detected on chromosomes 1p, 4, 10q, 13q, 17, and 19 with different techniques such as M-FISH, metaphase CGH, and allelotyping indicates that there is a selection pressure for dysregulation of unknown genes at these specific chromosomal loci.

9.3 SPECIFIC CELL CYCLE AND APOPTOTIC GENES DYSREGULATED IN CTCL

The p53 gene is commonly inactivated by mutations in a wide range of malignancies, but the significance varies for different tumor types. In CTCL studies have shown abnormal p53 expression particularly in late stages of MF,[16,17] and subsequently it was established that this is due to mutation of the p53 gene that appears to be restricted to stage IIB disease and/or large cell transformation, suggesting a role in disease progression.[18,19] P53 gene inactivation may occur in more than 40% of patients with tumor-stage MF. One study has shown evidence for UVB-specific mutations of the p53 gene, which might have important implications for the management of MF,[18] but these findings were not confirmed by a separate study.[19] P53 has a critical regulatory role through arrest of the cell cycle, allowing time for DNA repair, and the promotion of apoptosis. In NHLs, p53 mutations are associated with treatment resistance because most cancer therapies induce cell death by apoptotic mechanisms.[20] The cyclin-dependent kinase (CDK) inhibitors, p16 and p15, are also frequently inactivated in CTCL, but this usually occurs by promotor hypermethylation rather than mutation/deletion.[21,22] CDK inhibitors are also involved in regulation of the cell cycle, and their inactivation prevents cell cycle arrest. In contrast to p53, it appears that p15/16 gene inactivation may be present in both early and late stages of MF.[22]

Recent studies have shown rare Fas gene mutations in early stages of MF using microdissection methods, and there is also evidence for loss of Fas expression by tumor cells in late stages of MF,[23,24] which is consistent with high rates of loss of heterozygosity at the site of the Fas gene on 10q23.[7] Inactivation of the Fas gene would inhibit activation-induced cell death of malignant T cells and has also been detected in other types of NHLs.

Gene expression profiling in Sezary syndrome has identified two distinct gene expression signatures that have prognostic significance,[25] similar to recent studies in systemic diffuse large B-cell lymphomas.[26] These cDNA array studies in Sezary syndrome have also identified overexpression of genes specifically involved in Th2 development and dysregulation of genes involved in T-cell activation.[25] Preliminary cDNA array studies in MF have revealed abnormalities of tumor necrosis factor (TNF) signaling pathways and genes regulating apoptosis.[27]

The disruption of different apoptotic mechanisms would confer a survival advantage for tumor cells, allowing the accumulation of additional molecular abnormalities, and could also lead to treatment resistance, which is a common feature of late stages of CTCL. While p53, p15/16, and Fas gene abnormalities are also present in other types of NHL and solid malignancies,[28] their significance in CTCL should not be underestimated, and it is likely that other genes controlling both the cell cycle and apoptosis are also inactivated in CTCL. Future studies should establish the prevalence and prognostic significance of these abnormalities.

9.4   ABNORMALITIES OF T-CELL ACTIVATION IN CTCL

Both MF and Sezary syndrome are indolent tumors of mature CD4+ T cells, which usually express Th2 cytokines and chemokines. The IL-2 receptor is variably expressed, and tumor cells proliferate poorly. This is suggestive of defects in normal T-cell activation signaling pathways.

A high rate of genomic amplification of *JUNB* (19p13), a member of the Activator Protein-1 (AP-1) transcription factor complex, has recently been detected as part of an extensive array based CGH study of different oncogenes in CTCL.[29] These findings were confirmed with real-time PCR, which revealed that 24% of tumor samples showed *JUNB* gene amplification, while immunophenotypic studies confirmed JunB protein expression by tumor cells.[29] A recent cDNA microarray study has also detected consistent overexpression of JunB cDNA in Sezary syndrome.[25] These studies suggest that structural and numerical changes on chromosome 19 might be associated with copy number gains and overexpression of *JUNB* with

The AP-1 transcription factor complex is involved in the control of cell proliferation, differentiation, and apoptosis. This plethora of cellular effects is due to the complex structure of AP-1, which consists of a homo/heterodimer basic leucine-zipper DNA binding protein from the Jun, Fos, Maf, and/or ATF families. It is known that c-Jun promotes cell proliferation via induction of cyclin D1 and inhibition of p16, p21, and p53, while JunB antagonizes the effects of c-Jun via induction of p16 and repression of cyclin D1.[30] However a recent c-Jun knockout model suggests that, in the absence of c-Jun, JunB can also promote cell proliferation.[31] The precise function of this complex probably depends on the cell and tissue type and the structural content of the activated dimer, but AP-1 can function as both a positive and negative regulator of gene expression. Interactions with other transcription factors such as NFκB2, STAT3, and NFAT have been documented, and interestingly, constitutive activation of NFk B2 has also been detected in CTCL.[32,33] Aberrantly expressed c-Jun and JunB has also been detected in Hodgkin's disease,[34] and *JUNB* has been shown to induce CD30 expression in Hodgkin's disease, which can also be a feature of large cell transformation in MF.

AP-1 activity is regulated by a wide variety of stimuli, including growth factors, pro-inflammatory cytokines, and genotoxic stress via mitogen-activated protein kinase (MAPK) cascades such as the extracellular signal regulated kinase (ERK), c-Jun N-terminal kinase (JNK), and p38 MAPK cascades.[35] The activation of these MAP kinases are regulated by small G-proteins such as RHO proteins for the p38 MAPK and JNK kinases and activated oncogenes such as RAS and RAF for the ERK pathway. Interestingly, overexpression of RhoB has been detected recently in Sezary syndrome using cDNA microarrays,[25] and genomic amplification of RAF1 has also been detected in both MF and Sezary syndrome using array CGH and real-time PCR,[29] suggesting that abnormalities of MAP kinase pathways might also contribute to the dysregulation of AP-1 in CTCL. Recent studies have also established that disruption of these MAP kinase pathways occurs in leukemias and lymphomas including acute myeloid leukemia, Hodgkin's disease, and myeloma as well as adult T-cell leukemia-lymphoma.[36]

The specific role of AP-1 in T cells has only been partly determined. Early T-cell activation induced by binding of antigen with the TCR regulates the activity of various transcription factors in T-cells such as AP-1 and NFAT, which induce cytokine mediated T-cell activation, proliferation, and differentiation. Specifically, JunB binds to the IL-4 promotor and, in conjunction with c-Maf, promotes Th2 differentiation and expression of Th-2 cytokines.[30]

In contrast, late cytokine induced T-cell activation is mediated via signal transducers and activators of transcription (STAT) proteins, which have emerged as critical regulators of cellular proliferation, differentiation, and survival decisions.[37] Consequently, dysregulation of STAT function is a feature of many human malignancies.[38] Defects in the STAT signaling pathway have been implicated in CTCL, where studies have shown constitutive activation of STAT 3 in some MF and Sezary syndrome derived cell lines.[39,40]

The accumulation of activated T cells that proliferate poorly, as observed in Sezary syndrome, is reminiscent of the phenotype of both the IL-2 knockout and

TABLE 9.1
Summary of Molecular Abnormalities in Cutaneous T-Cell Lymphoma

Gene/Protein	Function	Mechanism	Disease
P53	Loss	Mutation/deletion	Mycosis fungoides (> stage IIB)/Sezary syndrome
P15/16	Loss	Methylation/deletion	Mycosis fungoides (> stage IIB)/Sezary syndrome
FAS	Loss	Mutation/deletion	Mycosis fungoides/Sezary syndrome
JUNB	Gain	Amplification	Mycosis fungoides/Sezary syndrome
hMLH1	Loss	Methylation	Mycosis fungoides (> stage IIB)
STATπ	Decreased	?	Sezary syndrome cell lines
STAT3	Increased	Constitutive activation	Sezary syndrome/mycosis fungoides cell lines
STAT5	Truncated	?	Sezary syndrome
BCL2	Loss	Deletion	Sezary syndrome
NFkB2	Gain	Mutation	Mycosis fungoides/cell lines

sively expressed as a C-terminally truncated isoform in the nuclei of normal peripheral T cells, while the full-length transcriptionally active form is expressed only after mitogenic stimulation.[41] Critically this activation-dependent STAT5 isoform expression is dysregulated in Sezary syndrome, with a concomitant loss of IL-2-induced STAT5-dependent gene expression.[41] The dysregulated, expression of C-terminal truncated STAT5 proteins in Sezary syndrome may be an important mechanism employed by malignant T cells to escape IL-2-induced apoptosis of activated T cells.

9.5   CONCLUSION

There is emerging evidence that genomic instability is a feature of CTCL and that specific chromosomal abnormalities are common. Future resolution of specific regions of chromosomal loss and gain is required to define putative genes that may be of fundamental pathogenetic importance in CTCL. Inactivation of pro-apoptotic genes and epigenetic changes are common as for other types of non-Hodgkin's lymphomas. In addition dysregulation of T-cell activation signaling pathways is a feature of MF and Sezary syndrome. This pattern of genetic and epigenetic abnormalities in CTCL provides the future rationale for the introduction of novel forms of therapy for this malignancy.

REFERENCES

1. Pileri, S., Pulford, K., Mori, S. et al. Frequent expression of the NPM-ALK chimeric fusion protein in anaplastic large cell lymphoma, lymphohistiocytic type. *Am. J. Pathol.* 150, 1207, 1997.
2. Rabbitts, T. Translocations, master genes, and differences between the origins of acute

3. Goldman, J. and Melo, J. Targeting the BCR-ABL tyrosine kinase in chronic myeloid leukaemia. *New England J. Med.* 344, 1084, 2001.
4. Mao, X., Lillington, D., Scarisbrick, J. et al. Molecular cytogenetic analysis of cutaneous T-cell lymphomas: identification of common genetic alterations in Sezary syndrome and mycosis fungoides. *Br. J. Dermatol.* 147, 464, 2002.
5. Mao, X., Orchard, G., Lillington, D. et al. Genetic alterations in primary cutaneous CD30+ anaplastic large cell lymphoma. *Genes, Chromosomes and Cancer* 37, 176, 2002.
6. Mao, X., Lillington, D., Czepulkowski, B. et al. Molecular cytogenetic characterization of Sezary syndrome. *Genes, Chromosomes and Cancer* 36, 250, 2003.
7. Scarisbrick, J., Woolford, A., Russell-Jones, R. et al. Loss of heterozygosity on 10q and microsatellite instability in advanced stages of primary cutaneous T-cell lymphoma and possible association with homozygous deletion of PTEN. *Blood* 95, 2937, 2000.
8. Scarisbrick, J., Mitchell, T., Calonje, E. et al. Microsatellite instability is associated with hypermethylation of the hMLHI gene and reduced expression in mycosis fungoides. *J. Invest. Dermatol.* 121, 894, 2003.
9. Thangavelu, M., Finn, W., Yelavarthi, K. et al. Recurring structural chromosomal abnormalities in peripheral blood lymphocytes of patients with mycosis fungoides/Sézary syndrome. *Blood* 89, 3371, 1997.
10. DeCoteau, J., Butmarc, J., Kinney, M. et al. The t(2;5) chromosomal translocation is not a common feature of primary cutaneous CD30+ lymphoproliferative disorders: comparison with large cell anaplastic lymphoma of nodal origin. *Blood* 87, 3437, 1996.
11. Kallionemi, A., Kallionemi, O.P., Suder, D. et al. Comparative genomic hybridization for molecular cytogenetic analysis of solid tumors. *Science* 258, 818, 1992.
12. Karenko, L., Kahkonen, M., Hyytinen, E. et al. Notable losses at specific regions of chromosome 10q and 13q in the Sézary syndrome detected by comparative genomic hybridization. *J. Invest. Dermatol.* 112, 392, 1999.
13. Scarisbrick, J.J., Woolford, A.J., Russell-Jones, R. et al. Allelotyping in mycosis fungoides and Sezary syndrome: common regions of allelic loss identified on 9p, 10q, and 17p. *J. Invest. Dermatol.* 117, 663, 2001.
14. Boni, R., Xin, H., Kamarashev, J. et al. Allelic deletion at 9p21-22 in primary cutaneous CD30+ large cell lymphoma. *J. Invest. Dermatol.* 115, 1104, 2000.
15. Boland, C., Thibodeau, S., Hamilton, S. et al. A National Cancer Institute workshop on microsatellite instability for cancer detection and familial predisposition: development of international criteria for the determination of microsatellite instability in colorectal cancer. *Cancer Res.* 58, 5248, 1998.
16. Lauritzen, A., Vejlsgaard, G., Hou-Jensen, K. et al. p53 protein expression in cutaneous T-cell lymphomas. *Br. J. Dermatol.* 133, 32, 1995.
17. McGregor, J., Dublin, E., Levison, D. et al. p53 immunoreactivity is uncommon in primary cutaneous lymphoma. *Br. J. Dermatol.* 132, 353, 1995.
18. McGregor, J., Crook, T., Fraser-Andrews, E. et al. Spectrum of p53 gene mutations suggests a possible role for ultraviolet radiation in the pathogenesis of advanced cutaneous lymphomas. *J. Invest. Dermatol.* 112, 317, 1999.
19. Marrogi, A., Khan, M., Vonderheid, E. et al. P53 tumour suppressor gene mutations in transformed cutaneous T-cell lymphoma: a study of 12 cases. *J. Cutaneous Pathol.* 26, 369, 1999.
20. Wilson, W., Teruya-Feldstein, J., Fest, T. et al. Relationship of p53, bcl-2, and tumor proliferation to clinical drug resistance in non-Hodgkin's lymphomas. *Blood* 89, 601,

21. Navas, I., Oritz-Romero, P., Villuendas, R. et al. P16 gene alterations are frequent in lesions of mycosis fungoides. *Am J. Pathol.* 156, 1565, 2000.
22. Scarisbrick, J.J., Woolford, A.J., Calonje, E. et al. Frequent abnormalities of the p15 and p16 genes in mycosis fungoides and Sezary syndrome. *J. Invest. Dermatol.* 118, 493, 2002.
23. Dereure, O., Levi, E., Vonderheid, E. et al. Infrequent Fas mutations but no Bax or p53 mutations in early mycosis fungoides: a possible mechanism for the accumulation of malignant T lymphocytes in the skin. *J. Invest. Dermatol.* 118, 949, 2002.
24. Zoi-Toli, O., Vermeer, M., De Vries, E. et al. Expression of Fas and Fas-ligand in primary cutaneous T-cell lymphoma (CTCL): association between lack of Fas expression and aggressive types of CTCL. *Br. J. Dermatol.* 143, 313, 2000.
25. Kari, L., Loboda, A., Nebozhyn, M. et al. Classification and prediction of survival in patients with the leukemic phase of cutaneous T cell lymphoma. *J. Exp. Med.* 197, 1477, 2003.
26. Rosenwald, A., Wright, G., Chan, W. et al. The use of molecular profiling to predict survival after chemotherapy for diffuse large B-cell lymphoma. *New England J. Med.* 346, 1937, 2002.
27. Tracey, L., Villuendas, R., Dotor, A. et al. Mycosis fungoides shows concurrent deregulation of multiple genes involved in the TNF signaling pathway: an expression profile study. *Blood* 102, 1042, 2003.
28. Gombart, A., Morosetti, R., Miller, C. et al. Deletions of the cyclin-dependant inhibitor genes p15 and p16 in non-Hodgkins lymphoma. *Blood* 86, 1534, 1995.
29. Mao, X., Orchard, G., Lillington, D. et al. Amplification and overexpression of JUNB is associated with primary cutaneous T-cell lymphomas. *Blood* 101, 1513, 2003.
30. Shaulian, E. and Karin, M. AP-1 in cell proliferation and survival. *Oncogene* 20, 2390, 2001.
31. Passegue, E., Jochum, W., Behrens, A. et al. JunB can substitute for Jun in mouse development and cell proliferation. *Nature Genetics* 30, 158, 2002.
32. Izban, K., Ergin, M., Qin, J.-Z. et al. Constitutive expression of NF-kB is a characteristic feature of mycosis fungoides: implications for apoptosis resistance and pathogenesis. *Hum. Pathol.* 31, 1482, 2000.
33. Migliazza, A., Lombardi, L., Rocchi, M. et al. Heterogenous chromosomal aberrations generate 3′ truncations of the NFKB2/lyt-10 gene in lymphoid malignancies. *Blood* 84, 3850, 1994.
34. Mathas, S., Hinz, M., Anagnostopoulos, I. et al. Aberrantly expressed c-Jun and JunB are a hallmark of Hodgkin lymphoma cells, stimulate proliferation and synergize with NF-kB. *EMBO* 21, 4104, 2002.
35. Rincon, M. MAP-kinase signaling pathways in T cells. *Curr. Opinion Immunol.* 13, 339, 2001.
36. Platinas L. MAP kinase signaling pathways and hematologic malignancies. *Blood* 101, 4667, 2003.
37. Levy, D. and Darnell, J. STATS: Transcriptional control and biological impact. Nature reviews: *Nat. Rev. Mol. Cell. Biol.*, 3, 651, 2002.
38. Bowman, T. and Jove, R. STAT proteins and cancer. *Cancer Control* 6, 615, 1999.
39. Zhang, Q., Nowak, I., Vonderheid, E. et al. Activation of Jak/STAT proteins involved in signal transduction pathway mediated by receptor for interleukin 2 in malignant T lymphocytes derived from cutaneous anaplastic large T-cell lymphoma and Sezary syndrome. *PNAS* 93, 9148, 1996.

40. Brender, C., Nielsen, M., Kaltoft, K. et al. STAT3-mediated constitutive expression of SOCS-3 in cutaneous T-cell lymphoma. *Blood* 97, 1056, 2001.

41. Mitchell, T.J., Whittaker, S.J., and John, S. Dysregulated expression of COOH-terminally truncated Stat5 and loss of IL-2 inducible Stat5-dependent gene expression in Sezary syndrome. *Cancer Res.* 63, 9048, 2003.

10 Treatment of Cutaneous T-Cell Lymphoma

Herschel S. Zackheim and Mohammed Kashani-Sabet

CONTENTS

TABLE 10.1
Tumor Node Metastasis (TNM) Classification for Cutaneous T-Cell Lymphoma

T: Skin
    T1: Patches and/or plaques covering <10% of skin surface
    T2a: Patches covering 10% of skin surface
    T2b: Plaques covering 10% skin surface
    T3: Tumor stage
    T4: Generalized erythroderma (80% skin surface)
N: Lymph nodes
    N0: No clinically abnormal peripheral lymph nodes, pathology negative for CTCL
    N1: Clinically abnormal lymph nodes, pathology negative for CTCL
    N2: No clinically abnormal peripheral lymph nodes, pathology positive for CTCL
    N3: Clinically abnormal peripheral lymph nodes, pathology positive for CTCL
B: Peripheral blood
    B0: No evidence of blood involvement by CTCL
    B1: Evidence of blood involvement by CTCL
M: Visceral organs
    M0: No visceral organ involvement
    M1: Visceral organ involvement (confirmed by pathology)

Note: CTCL, cutaneous T-cell lymphoma.

Source: Kashani-Sabet, M., McMillan, A., and Zackheim, H.S. *J. Am. Acad. Dermatol.* 45, 700, 2001.

As is generally true for malignancies, treatment of cutaneous T-cell lymphoma (CTCL; mycosis fungoides [MF]/Sezary syndrome [SS]) varies with disease stage. Classification of CTCL according to stage[1] is presented in Tables 10.1 and 10.2. The clinical features of CTCL are described in Chapter 2. Fung et al.[2] recently authored a comprehensive review of CTCL and other cutaneous lymphomas.

10.1 TOPICAL THERAPY

10.1.1 TOPICAL CORTICOSTEROIDS

At the University of California, San Francisco (UCSF) our first-line treatment for patch-stage MF is class I topical corticosteroids (CSs).[3] Clobetasol 0.05% is usually prescribed because it appears to be as effective as other class I topical CSs and is available as a generic, which makes it generally acceptable to insurance carriers,

Clobetasol is usually prescribed as a cream because of patient preference — it is less messy than the ointment. However, if it appears to be less effective than expected or if it causes irritation, then the ointment is prescribed. The patient is instructed to rub the preparation in *vigorously* twice daily. Vigorous application is necessary to achieve maximum penetration and, therefore, effectiveness. Patients

TABLE 10.2
Staging Classification for
Cutaneous T-Cell Lymphoma

IA	T1	N0	M0
IB	T2a	N0	M0
IIA	T1,2a	N1	M0
IIB	T2b	N0,1	M0
IIIA	T3	N0,1	M0
IIIB	T4	N0,1	M0
IVA	T1–4	N2,3	M0
IVB	T1–4	N0–3	M1

Source: Kashani-Sabet, M., McMillan, A., and Zackheim, H.S. *J. Am. Acad. Dermatol.* 45, 700, 2001.

are told to ignore any pharmacist's instructions or package inserts that call for applying the preparation lightly or sparingly.

Preparations are to be applied twice daily, without interruption, until the patient is told to stop or to decrease the frequency of applications. There is generally no limitation on the total area treated with the possible exception of elderly, frail patients who might be at risk for the development of adrenal suppression. Patients are told to disregard the package insert, which calls for limitation of periods of treatment and amount used (Temovate[R]; GlaxoSmithKline). Lesions on the extremities are often treated with plastic film occlusion at night, in addition to daily applications without occlusion.

Elderly patients with widespread lesions are often treated with the medium strength 0.1% triamcinolone cream or ointment under plastic suit occlusion two or three times weekly. The preparation is usually applied in the early evening, left on for about 3 hours or at least until a good sweat is induced, and then washed off prior to going to bed. Patients are not encouraged to sleep in the suit, as they may become cold and clammy, which can predispose them to upper respiratory infection.

Although morning serum cortisol levels were obtained in the early phase of this study, they are not now obtained routinely except in elderly, frail patients with extensive lesions. In this regard we follow the recommendation of Bromberg[4] that the adrenal function of patients receiving exogenous steroids need not be tested except when there are clear-cut clinical indications. None of our patients have shown clinical signs of adrenal insufficiency such as fatigue, anorexia, and weight loss.

Seventy-nine patients with patch-stage (75 patients) or plaque-stage (4 patients) CTCL were treated with topical CSs. The following maximum response rates were obtained: stage T1 (<10% skin involved) complete response (CR) 63%; partial response (PR) (50% improvement) 31%; total response (TR) 94%; stage T2 (10% skin involved) CR 25%, PR 57%, TR 82%. Only 3 of 51 stage T1 patients and 1 of 31 stage T2 patients had plaque-stage disease. Of the 3 patients with stage T1 plaque-stage disease, 1 was in partial remission, 1 was stable, and 1 had progressive

TABLE 10.3
Mycosis Fungoides Response to Topical Corticosteroids (Median Follow-Up 9 Months)

Stage	No.	Maximum Response, No. (%)					Last Status, No. (%)				
		CR	PR	SD	PD	TR	CR	PR	SD	PD	TR
T1	51	32(63)	16(31)	3(6)	0(0)	48(94)	19(37)	22(43)	8(16)	2(4)	41(80)
T2	28	7(25)	16(57)	5(18)	0(0)	23(82)	5(18)	14(50)	6(21)	3(11)	19(68)

Note: CR, complete remission; PR, partial remission; SD, stable disease; PD, progressive disease; TR, total response (CR + PR).

Source: Zackheim, H.S., Kashani-Sabet, M., and Amin, S. *Arch. Dermatol.* 134, 949, 1998. With permission.

disease at the last examination. The stage T2 plaque-stage patient developed progressive disease.

At their last visit (median follow-up 9 months), 37% of stage T1 patients were in complete remission and 43% were in partial remission for a total response rate of 80%. Of the stage T2 patients, 18% were in complete remission and 50% were in partial remission for a total response rate of 68% (Table 10.3).

Side effects were minor; the most common were purpura and irritant dermatitis, both occurring in 10% to 20% of the patients. Striae and atrophy were seen in a few patients. The atrophy was reversible but striae were persistent.

As of the present writing, more than 200 patients with patch-stage MF have been treated at UCSF with topical CSs, mostly clobetasol. The results continue to be very favorable and are essentially similar to those reported in our 1998 study. Topical CSs are readily available by prescription, and patient acceptance is high. Topical CSs remain our first-line treatment for patch-stage MF.

10.1.2 TOPICAL MECHLORETHAMINE

Topical mechlorethamine (MCH) is widely used in the treatment of MF. MCH is commonly referred to as "nitrogen mustard." However, MCH is but one of several nitrogen mustard compounds used as chemotherapeutic agents; these include melphalan, cyclophosphamide, ifosfamide, and chlorambucil.[5] Nitrogen mustards exert their antineoplastic effect by means of alkylation. All alkylating agents are potentially mutagenic and carcinogenic, as well as cytotoxic. MCH is used systemically mostly as part of combination chemotherapy for Hodgkin's lymphoma.

MCH was first reported by Sipos in Hungarian as topical therapy for MF in 1956. The first English language report was that by Haserick in 1959.[5] MCH is still probably the most widely used topical therapy for patch/plaque MF. MCH can be used topically as an aqueous solution or as an ointment.[5] MCH comes as a vial containing 10 mg MCH and 90 mg sodium chloride as Mustargen (Merck). The aqueous solution is prepared by dissolving the MCH powder (and sodium applied to the total body surface; however, intertriginous areas are treated lightly, and the face and genitals are spared unless they have active lesions. Some investigators treat only involved areas. The maximum response usually occurs within 3 to 6 months.

MCH ointment is prepared by dissolving one 10 mg vial of MCH in 10 ml of 95% (absolute) alcohol, then mixing this solution with an anhydrous ointment base such as white petrolatum USP or Aquaphor®. The usual concentration is 10 mg/100g ointment base (10 mg%). Applications are made daily similarly to the technique used for MCH solution. Time to clearing (6 to 12 months) is usually longer than is required for the solution.

With both the solution and ointment, maintenance therapy after clearing is often continued daily for varying periods followed by tapering doses. However, some physicians do not use maintenance therapy and may retreat only in the event of relapse.

In this regard, the report of Volden et al.[6] is relevant. Two patients developed infiltrated plaques during maintenance therapy after complete clearing and were then resistant to topical MCH. However, after rest periods of 4 and 6 months they again were responsive. The investigators favor intermittent therapy to be used only in the event of a relapse.

Ramsay and coauthors[7] treated 107 patients with patch/plaque-stage MF with topical aqueous solutions of MCH. CR was obtained in 67% of those with less than 10% skin involvement (stage T1) after 1 year, and in 40% of those with more than 10% involvement (stage T2). The median time to achieve CR was 4.4 months for stage T1 patients and 20 months for stage T2 patients. Delayed hypersensitivity reactions occurred in 58% of the patients. However, because of successful topical desensitization, only 1 patient had to discontinue treatment. However, 10% of the patients developed an immediate-type urticarial reaction and had to discontinue MCH due to the possibility of anaphylaxis. No increase in secondary cutaneous malignancies was seen, with a median follow-up of 3.3 years.

Kim et al.[8] recently reported an update of the Stanford experience in the treatment of MF with topical MCH. Of 203 patients who were treated, 68% were treated only with MCH. These were generally patients with patch or thin-plaque disease. In this group, freedom from progression exceeded 90%. Most of the patients were treated with the ointment-based preparation since the 1980s. There was no statistically significant difference in efficacy or survival between the ointment versus the aqueous solution.

The most common side effect was irritant or allergic contact dermatitis. With the ointment preparation, a quarter of the patients experienced irritant reactions. These were usually mild. Nearly all patents were able to continue therapy by decreasing the frequency of application or the concentration. Up to two thirds of the patients using the aqueous solution developed contact hypersensitivity reactions compared to fewer than 10% of those using the ointment preparation. Most patients were desensitized by reduction of the concentration followed by gradual escalation.

Nonmelanoma skin cancers occurred in only 2 (1%) of the 139 patients who used MCH monotherapy. However, these occurred at sites (face) not treated with MCH. One of the 203 patients had melanoma. He was elderly, with Fitzpatrick skin

The authors conclude that topical MCH is an effective and safe therapy for patients with limited or extensive patch and/or plaque-stage disease (T1–T2).

10.1.3 TOPICAL CARMUSTINE/BISCHLOROETHYLNITROSOUREA

Carmustine (also named BCNU, for bischloroethylnitrosourea) is a nitrosourea type alkylating compound used in cancer chemotherapy. Its principal indication is for central nervous system malignancies. Zackheim first reported the topical use of BCNU for CTCL in 1972,[9] and since then there have been a number of studies by Zackheim and co-workers on topical BCNU for CTCL (see later).

BCNU (BiCNU; Bristol-Myers Squibb Oncology/Virology) can be used either as a solution or as an ointment. As a solution, the BCNU powder is first dissolved in 95% ethanol. This appears to be stable for at least 1 year when refrigerated. For extensive lesions (over 50% of the body surface), the contents of one vial of BiCNU (100 mg) are dissolved in 50 ml of 95% or absolute ethanol. This yields a concentration of 2 mg/ml. Then 5 ml of this stock solution (10 mg BCNU) is diluted with 60 ml water. Only involved areas are treated. If less than half of the body surface is involved, then 2.5 ml of the stock solution is diluted with 30 ml water. The solution is best applied with a 2-inch nylon brush or gauze pads. Plastic or latex gloves should be worn. Limited areas (less than 3% of the body surface) can be treated cautiously with the undiluted alcoholic stock solution (2 mg/ml) once daily using a cotton-tipped applicator.

BCNU ointment is prepared by mixing an alcoholic solution of BCNU with white petrolatum USP. The ointment appears to be stable for at least 1 year when refrigerated. However, any ointment that turns brown (indicating oxidation) should be discarded. Most commonly a concentration of 20 mg/100 g ointment base (20 mg%) is used. Applications are made once daily to involved areas only. Protective gloves should be used.

Zackheim et al.[10] in 1990 reported response rates in 109 patients with patch/plaque MF treated with BCNU solution. In patients with less than 10% skin involvement (T1), CR was obtained in 86%, and PR in 12%, for a TR of 98%. For those with 10% or more involvement (T2), the corresponding responses were CR 47%, PR 37%, and TR 84%.

In 1995 Ramsay et al.[11] reported results in 188 patients with patch/plaque MF treated with BCNU solution. Because of the long-term nature of the study, responses were reported in terms of freedom from treatment failure (FFTF). Patients were followed for up to 218 days. The median FFTF period for T1 patients was not reached. For T2 patients, the median FFTF was 86 months. At 36 months, 91% of T1 patients and 62% of T2 patients had not failed treatment. Some degree of erythema, simulating a sunburn, was experienced by most patients. Body folds were most often involved. Severe reactions were often accompanied by skin tenderness and were also often followed by telangiectasia. The telangiectasia lasted from several months to as long as 11 years; however, it was not accompanied by changes indicating premalignant change such as hyperkeratosis. Mild leukopenia (lowest WBC 2700/mm^3) occurred in 3.7% of the patients. Allergic reactions were limited to the skin and occurred in less than 10% of the patients. No skin cancers related to BCNU treatment were noted.

Experience with BCNU ointment is considerably less than that with the solution, and a report of a series of patients has not been published. It is our impression that the ointment causes milder cutaneous reactions than the solution but is less effective. It is easier to use than the solution but is messier.

Complete blood counts should be obtained at the start of and once monthly during treatment for both the solution and ointment. Blood chemistries may be advisable every 3 months, although we have seen no alterations related to BCNU therapy. Treatment should be stopped if severe cutaneous reactions occur. Topical corticosteroids or other anti-inflammatory measures should be used.

10.1.4 Topical Bexarotene

Bexarotene (a "rexinoid") is a recently introduced retinoid. It is selective for the retinoid X receptors (RXR) and is used both orally and topically. Breneman et al.[12] treated 67 patients with early stage CTCL with varying concentrations of bexarotene gel in a phase 1 and 2 trial. Most patients tolerated the 1% gel twice daily. The median projected time to response was 20.1 weeks. The complete response rate was 21% and the overall response rate was 63%. Local erythema and/or irritation occurred in 87% of the patients but were mostly mild to moderate.

More recently, Heald et al.[13] conducted a multinational open-label phase III trial of 1% bexarotene gel in 50 patients with refractory patch/plaque MF. The overall response rates for the Physicians Global Assessment, Composite Assessment of Index Lesion severity, and primary end point classification were 44%, 46%, and 54%, respectively. The most common adverse events were irritant dermatitis, pruritus, burning at application site, and skin disorder. There were no serious treatment-related adverse events. The investigators conclude that bexarotene gel was generally well tolerated and demonstrated substantial efficacy.

10.2 PHOTOTHERAPY

10.2.1 Broadband UVB

Broadband UVB (280 to 350 nm) has well-documented efficacy for patch-stage MF.[14] Resnick and Vonderheid[15] reported long-term (15-year) follow-up of 31 patients with patch and early plaque-stage MF treated at home with broadband UVB. CR occurred in 23 patients (74%) with a maximum duration of response from 5 months to more than 15 years (the median was 51 months). Only 3 patients required treatment for actinic keratoses, and none had squamous cell carcinoma. Ramsay et al.[16] treated 37 patients with early stage CTCL with broadband UVB. Approximately three fourths of the patients either started UVB therapy at home or changed to home treatment after starting therapy in an outpatient hospital setting. Approximately one fourth of the patients were treated only as outpatients. Eighty-three percent of 30 patients with patch-stage disease achieved CR, whereas none of 4 patients with plaque-stage lesions achieved CR.

10.2.2 Narrowband UVB

In recent years a number of reports have attested to the effectiveness of narrowband UVB (311–312 nm) for early stage MF. Hofer et al.[17] reported results in 20 patients with either small plaque parapsoriasis (14 patients) or patch-stage MF (6 patients). In 19 patients lesions cleared completely after a mean of 20 treatments within 5 to 10 weeks. However, local relapses occurred in all patients within a mean time of 6 months (the range was 2 to 15 months).

Clark et al.[18] reported 8 patients with patch-stage MF who were treated with narrowband UVB. Complete clearance was achieved in 6 patients in a mean of 9 weeks, and 4 patients have had prolonged remissions (with a mean duration of 20 months). The largest series of MF patients treated with narrowband UVB was reported by Gathers et al.[19] Twenty-four patients with patch-stage MF were treated. Mean follow-up period was 29.0 weeks. CR was obtained in 13 patients (54.2%), PR in 29.2%, and no response in 16.7%. Four patients with CR relapsed (30.8%), with a mean time to relapse of 12.5 weeks.

10.2.3 UVA1

Recent reports have documented responses of patients with CTCL to UVA1 (340–400 nm) therapy. Plettenberg et al.[20] treated 3 patients with early stage MF with UVA1. In all patients complete clearance was obtained after 16 to 20 exposures. von Kobyletski et al.[21] treated a 68-year-old man with progressive erythrodermic CTCL with UVA1. Treatments were given five times a week for 3 weeks. At each session 60 J/cm^2 was applied for a cumulative dose of 900 J/cm^2. After 3 weeks, the skin had almost normalized, and this was sustained during a follow-up of 8 weeks. Stander and Schwarz[22] treated a 36-year-old male with limited patch-stage MF with UVA1 at increasing doses of UVA1 of up to 80 J/cm^2 given five times per week. After 67 treatments delivered within 4 months, the lesions had completely disappeared. A biopsy was taken from a previously involved area. This still revealed typical changes of MF, including a dense dermal infiltrate. Gene rearrangement studies indicated a monoclonal infiltrate. In view of this finding, posttreatment biopsies should be routinely obtained in patients treated with UVA1, at least until the value of UVA1 in the treatment of CTCL is well established. The largest series of MF patients treated with UVA1 is that of Zane et al.[23] Thirteen patients with MF (8 with extensive plaque-stage MF, 4 with tumor-stage MF but without subcutaneous involvement, and 1 with erythrodermic MF) were treated with UVA1. Daily exposures of 100 J/cm^2 were given five times weekly. The mean cumulative dose was 2148.5 J/cm^2 with a mean of 21.9 exposures. The irradiations required 42 minutes but were well tolerated. Three of the tumor-stage patients had complete clearing of the exposed lesions, and 1 had partial clearing. The 1 patient with erythrodermic MF experienced complete remission of the exposed lesions.

It is apparent that results with UVA1 in the treatment of MF are encouraging but that further experience is needed to better evaluate the potential usefulness of UVA1 in the management of that disease.

10.2.4 PSORALENS PLUS UVA (PUVA)

Psoralens plus UVA (PUVA) combines the use of a photosensitizing agent (psoralen) with UVA (320 to 400 nm). Patients ingest 5- or 8-methoxypsoralen 1.5 to 2 hours prior to exposure to UVA. Treatments are given two to three times a week until maximum improvement is obtained.

PUVA has had an established role in the treatment of CTCL since it was introduced by Gilchrest et al. in 1976.[24] Results of treatment as of 1995 were summarized by Herrmann et al.[14] Complete response rates ranged from 76% to 90% in early stage (patch/plaque) disease. Although 59% of tumor-stage patients achieved CR, many required additional radiation therapy. Erythrodermic patients may respond well, but the relapse rate is high (82%). Because the relapse rate for all stages is considerable, maintenance therapy is recommended. The most common acute side effects, affecting 7% to 10% of patients, are burning/erythema and pruritus. The most common chronic complications, involving 3% to 5% of patients, are squamous and basal cell carcinoma, solar lentigo, and keratoacanthoma. More recently prolonged treatment with PUVA has been confirmed as a risk factor for the development of melanoma.[25]

Diederen et al.[26] recently compared narrowband UVB (NBUVB) with PUVA in a retrospective study of 56 patients with early stage MF. The total response rate was 100% in both groups. The mean relapse-free interval was 24.5 months for patients treated with NBUVB and 22.8 months for patients treated with PUVA. The follow-up periods were too short to permit a comparison of long-term sequelae. Patients treated with NBUVB had fewer side effects than the PUVA-treated patients. The investigators recommend NBUVB as initial therapy and switching to PUVA if results are unsatisfactory.

Thomsen et al.[27] demonstrated that patients treated with combination therapy of PUVA and the retinoids etretinate and isotretinoin required fewer PUVA sessions and a lower UVA dosage. In a recent report the combination of PUVA and the novel retinoid bexarotene had an overall favorable effect in a series of 5 patients with advanced CTCL.[28] PUVA has also been used in combination with interferon alfa-2a in advanced CTCL. Results were described as highly effective[29] or useful.[30]

10.2.5 EXTRACORPOREAL PHOTOPHERESIS

Extracorporeal photopheresis (ECP) is a modification of PUVA in which, after the ingestion of psoralens, circulating mononuclear cells, instead of the skin, are exposed to UVA. Treatment is usually in 2-day cycles, once monthly, for a minimum of 6 months. The best results have been obtained in early to moderately advanced erythrodermic MF.[31] Responses in patients with plaque and tumor-stage MF[32] and in erythrodermic patients with evidence of a circulating T-cell clone[33] are not impressive. Gottlieb et al.[34] treated 28 patients with mostly advanced-stage CTCL with ECP alone. Nine of these patients went on to receive combination therapy with IFN-α and, in some cases, other agents. Among these 9 patients, 5 had an enhanced response as compared to ECP treatment alone. Suchin et al.[35] summarized a 14-year experience in 47 patients with CTCL treated with ECP. Thirty-one of the patients received a combination of ECP plus one or more immunostimulatory agents including IFN-α, IFN-, sagramostim, or systemic retinoids. The group that received combination therapy had better response rates and overall survival than those receiving ECP monotherapy.

10.3 IONIZING RADIATION

10.3.1 ORTHOVOLTAGE RADIATION

In years past orthovoltage radiation was widely used in the management of patients with widespread, infiltrated plaques, or tumors. Although this was generally effective, the long-term complications such as cutaneous atrophy, telangiectasia, squamous cell carcinoma and other cutaneous malignancies was a distinct disadvantage. Orthovoltage radiation has largely been replaced by electron beam (EB) therapy.

10.3.2 ELECTRON BEAM RADIATION

EB radiation is used to treat tumors and deeply infiltrated plaques.

10.3.2.1 Local EB Therapy

Patients with localized or small numbers of deeply infiltrated plaques or tumors are often treated with local EB. As a rule, treatment is highly effective with prolonged remissions and minimal side effects.

10.3.2.2 Total Skin Electron Beam Therapy

Total skin EB (TSEB) therapy is indicated for patients with widespread infiltrated plaques and tumors. Some physicians also use TSEB to treat early stage disease and erythroderma.[36] The Stanford technique is probably the most widely used.[37]

10.3.2.2.1 Technique

The treatment consists of 36 treatment visits in 9 weeks, with 4 consecutive visits per week. The patient is treated standing at 6 different positions. Two-hundred rads (2 Gy) is given to the skin surface over a 2-day cycle for a total of 3600 rad (36 Gy).

Treatment is by a linear accelerator producing 6-MeV electrons at 4 m from the patient. Boosts are required to the perineum, soles, tumors, and thick plaques.

10.3.2.2.2 Sequelae: Short-term

The most common short-term sequelae (all reversible) are erythema, hyperpigmentation, alopecia, nail dystrophy, and peripheral edema with possible bullae.

10.3.2.2.3 Sequelae: Long-term

With the schedule as described, significant long-term (6 months) effects are minimal, although occasional patients may have some degree of permanent scalp alopecia. Infertility may occur in men, related to perineum boost.

TABLE 10.4
Therapy for Cutaneous T-Cell Lymphoma

Modality	Stage	Topical	Photo	PhotChem	Radiation	Oral	SC	IM	IV
Corticosteroids	T1–2	X							
Mechlorethamine	T1–2	X							
Carmustine	T1–2	X							
UVB	T1–2		X						
PUVA	T1–2			X					
Photopheresis	T2–4			X					
Methotrexate	T2–4					X	X	X	X
Bexarotene gel	T1–4	X							
IFNα	T1–4						X		
Electron beam	T1–4				X				
Orthovoltage radiation	T1–3				X				
Denileukin diftitox	T2–4								X
Other chemotherapy	T2–4					X	X		X X

Source: Fung, M.A. et al. *J. Am. Acad. Dermatol.* 46, 325, 2002. With permission.

Repeated courses of TSEB may be given, although these are usually at a lower dose than that given for the first course.[36] As a rule, other therapies are tried before repeating TSEB.

10.4 SYSTEMIC THERAPY

10.4.1 LOW-DOSE METHOTREXATE

Although low-dose methotrexate (MTX) has been widely used for MF for many years, such use is poorly documented. Since the report of Wright et al.[38] in 1964 involving 16 patients, there has been no published series of patients treated with low-dose MTX with the exception of the study of Zackheim et al.[39] involving 29 patients with erythrodermic CTCL. However, Zackheim et al.[40] very recently documented long-term experience with low-dose MTX in the management of patch/plaque and tumor-stage MF in a cohort of 69 patients followed for up to 201 months.

MTX was given once weekly, mostly orally, at a usual maximum dose of 50 mg, occasionally 75 mg. The median weekly dose was approximately 25 mg. The great majority (60) of the patients were patch/plaque-stage T2 (10% skin involved). Of these, 7 (12%) achieved complete remission and 13 (22%) achieved partial remission for a total response rate of 20 of 60 (33%). The median time to treatment failure was 15 months. Patients with predominantly patch-stage disease had a superior response rate and a longer period of time to treatment failure as compared to those with predominantly plaque-stage disease. Only 1 of 7 patients with tumor-stage lesions responded. Side effects caused treatment failure in 6 (9%) of the total cohort of 69 patients. Low-dose MTX may be of value in the management of a subset of patients with patch/plaque MF resistant to other therapies.

10.4.2 Interferon-α (IFN-α)

There has been considerable experience with IFN-α in the treatment of CTCL. IFN-α is given subcutaneously and can be self-administered. The usual starting dose is 3 million units (MU) three times per week. This is gradually escalated as needed and tolerated. The principal toxicities are malaise, mostly in older patients, and low-grade fever. IFN-α is generally well tolerated.

Results as of 1995 were summarized by Olsen and Bunn.[41] In a meta-analysis of 14 studies involving 207 patients using IFN-α as a single agent, the overall response rate was 54%. When used in combination with other agents, the most favorable results were obtained in combination with PUVA. However, comparisons of different combinations is hazardous because these were not prospective, randomized trials, and there may have been considerable differences in the proportion of patients with early and advanced-stage disease treated with the different combinations.

Since the Olsen and Bunn report, the largest series of patients treated with IFN-α as monotherapy is that of Jumbou et al.[42] A total of 51, mostly advanced-stage, patients were followed for a mean follow-up period of 43.4 months. The overall response rate was 66.7%. The combination of IFN-α-2a and PUVA was used by Chiarion-Sileni et al.[43] in 63 patients. After dose escalation for 1 month, patients received 12 MU TIW for up to 1 year. Complete or partial responses were obtained in 51 patients (74.6%). Stadler et al.[44] compared IFN-α plus acitretin versus IFN-α plus PUVA in a prospective randomized trial involving 82 stage I and II CTCL patients. The IFN + PUVA group with 70% complete remissions was significantly superior to the IFN + acitretin group with 38.1% complete remissions. Wollina et al.[45] treated 14 patients with stage II CTCL with IFN-α plus ECP. After 1 year, the total response rate was 46%. Only one of 4 patients with tumor-stage (IIb) disease responded.

10.4.3 Bexarotene

A recent addition to the therapeutic options for both early and advanced-stage CTCL is the novel retinoid bexarotene. Bexarotene is a rexinoid, the first RXR-selective retinoid agonist to be studied in humans. Bexarotene can be administered orally or topically. Topical bexarotene is discussed in section 10.1.4 of this chapter.

In a multicenter study[46] oral bexarotene was given to patients with refractory early-stage CTCL at doses of 300 mg/m^2/d. The drug was well tolerated and effective in 15 (54%) of 28 patients. The most frequent adverse events included hypertriglyceridemia (associated rarely with pancreatitis), hypercholesterolemia, hypothyroidism, and headache. Duvic et al.[47] evaluated oral bexarotene in 94 patients with advanced-stage CTCL. At a dose of 300 mg/m^2/d the total response rate was 45%. Adverse events were similar to those observed in patients with early-stage disease.

10.4.4 Denileukin Diftitox

Denileukin diftitox is a recently introduced systemic agent for the treatment of interleukin (IL)-2. Olsen et al.[48] treated 71 patients of whom 63% had tumor-stage or greater disease. Overall, 30% of the patients had an objective response. The most frequent side effects were constitutional symptoms, gastrointestinal disorders, and infection. The vascular leak syndrome occurred in approximately one fourth of the patients. Five patients with the vascular leak syndrome required hospitalization for management of complications including pulmonary edema and renal insufficiency.

10.4.5 SINGLE AGENT AND COMBINATION CHEMOTHERAPY

Systemic chemotherapy for CTCL as of 1995 was reviewed by Rosen and Foss.[49] A wide variety of single agents and combinations have been used. Long-term remissions or cures were rarely seen. There have been a number of studies since. Sarris et al.[50] treated 15 patients with MF or SS (MF/SS), 3 with anaplastic large cell lymphoma (ALCL), and 2 with peripheral T-cell lymphoma with the lipophilic antifolate trimetrexate. For patients with MF/SS the response rate was 0% for those with histologically indolent disease and 50% for those with evidence of large cell transformation.

Bouwhuis et al.[51] reviewed results with 2-chlorodeoxyadenosine in 6 patients with late-stage SS. Two patients responded well to treatment. Four patients either had a partial response (1 patient) or had no response (3 patients). Mortality was 50% and was mostly due to infectious complications. Wollina et al.[52] treated 10 patients with relapsing or recalcitrant CTCL with pegylated liposomal doxorubicin. Eight patients achieved complete or partial remission. Wollina et al.[53] reported responses of 3 patients with tumor-stage CTCL to liposomal daunorubicin. One patient obtained a complete and 2 a partial response. Zinzani et al.[54] treated 44 previously treated patients with MF and 14 patients with peripheral T-cell lymphoma limited to the skin with gemcitabine, a novel pyrimidine antimetabolite, given intravenously. Complete or partial responses were achieved in 70.5% of the patients. Treatment was well tolerated. Argiris et al.[55] treated 12 patients with advanced CTCL with intravenous infusions of 9-aminocamptothecin. The response rate was low. The rate of complicated neutropenia and septic deaths was unacceptable.

Fierro et al.[56] treated 25 patients with advanced-stage CTCL with the combination of etoposide, idarubicin, cyclophosphamide, vincristine, prednisone, and bleomycin (VICOP-B). The overall response rate was 80%. The MF response rate was 84% with a median duration of 8.7 months. None of the SS patients responded. The authors conclude that VICOP-B is effective and feasible as first-line chemotherapy in advanced MF, with or without extracutaneous involvement. Scarisbrick et al.[57] treated 12 patients with CTCL (9 with erythrodermic CTCL and 3 with tumor-stage MF) with combination intravenous fludarabine and cyclophosphamide. The results indicate that the combination may be of clinical benefit but does not affect survival.

10.4.6 ANTIBODY AND TRANSPLANTATION THERAPY

A phase 2 study of alemtuzumab (anti-CD52 monoclonal antibody) was made by Lundin et al.[58] to treat 22 patients with advanced MF/SS. The overall response rate was 55%. The effect was better on erythroderma than on plaques or tumors. All serious infectious adverse events occurred in heavily pretreated patients. Guitart et cell transplantation after cytoreductive chemotherapy and total-body irradiation. Complete and sustained remission was achieved in 2 patients. Soligo et al.[60] performed nonmyeloablative transplantation of allogeneic stem cells in 3 patients with advanced CTCL. All patients achieved complete remissions but experienced a high prevalence of infections including one fatality. Russell-Jones et al.[61] performed autologous peripheral blood stem cell transplantation in 9 patients with tumor-stage MF, 4 of whom had lymph node involvement. Complete remission was achieved in 8 patients but was short-lived in 4. Conditioning was achieved with total skin EB, total body irradiation, and chemotherapy.

10.4.7 NOVEL AGENTS

Novel agents in the management of CTCL have been reviewed by Kuzel et al.[62]

REFERENCES

1. Kashani-Sabet, M., McMillan, A., and Zackheim, H.S. A modified staging classification for cutaneous T-cell lymphoma. *J. Am. Acad. Dermatol.* 45, 700, 2001.
2. Fung, M.A. et al. Practical evaluation and management of cutaneous lymphoma. *J. Am. Acad. Dermatol.* 46, 325, 2002.
3. Zackheim, H.S., Kashani-Sabet, M., and Amin, S. Topical corticosteroids for mycosis Fungoides: experience in 79 patients. *Arch. Dermatol.* 134, 949, 1998.
4. Bromberg, J.S. Adrenal insufficiency. *New Engl. J. Med.* 336, 1105, 1997.
5. Zackheim, H.S. Topical and intralesional chemotherapeutic agents, in *Comprehensive Dermatologic Drug Therapy*, Wolverton, S.E., Ed., W.B. Saunders, Philadelphia, 2001, chap. 29.
6. Volden, G., Molin, L., and Thomsen, K. Topical mechlorethamine therapy for mycosis fungoides. Proposed schedule to overcome drug resistance. *Arch. Dermatol.* 118, 138, 1982.
7. Ramsay, D.L., Halperin, P., and Zeleniuch-Jacquotte, J.A. Topical mechlorethamine therapy for early stage mycosis fungoides. *J. Am. Acad. Dermatol.* 19, 684, 1988.
8. Kim, Y.H. et al. Topical nitrogen mustard in the management of mycosis fungoides. Update of the Stanford experience. *J. Am. Acad. Dermatol.* 139, 165, 2003.
9. Zackheim, H.S. Treatment of mycosis fungoides with topical nitrosourea compounds. *J. Am. Acad. Dermatol.* 106, 177, 1972.
10. Zackheim, H.S., Epstein, E.H., Jr., and Crain, W.R. Topical carmustine (BCNU) for cutaneous T-cell lymphoma: a 15 year experience in 143 patients. *J. Am. Acad. Dermatol.* 22, 802, 1990.
11. Ramsay, D.L., Meller, J.A., and Zackheim, H.S. Topical treatment of early cutaneous T-cell lymphoma. *Hematol./Oncol. Clin. North Am.* 9, 1031, 1995.
12. Breneman, D. et al. Phase 1 and 2 trial of bexarotene gel for skin-directed treatment of patients with cutaneous T-cell lymphoma. *Arch. Dermatol.* 138, 325, 2002.
13. Heald, P. et al. Topical bexarotene therapy for patients with refractory or persistent early-stage cutaneous T-cell lymphoma: Results of the phase III clinical trial. *J. Am. Acad. Dermatol.* 49, 801, 2003.
14. Herrman, J.J., Roenigk, H.H., Jr, and Honigsman, H.H. Ultraviolet radiation for treatment of cutaneous T-cell lymphoma. *Hematol./Oncol. Clin. North Am.* 9, 1077, 1995.

15. Resnick, K.S. and Vonderheid, E.C. Home UV phototherapy of early mycosis fungoides: long-term follow-up observations in thirty-one patients. *J. Am. Acad. Dermatol.* 29, 73, 1993.
16. Ramsay, D.L. et al. Ultraviolet-B phototherapy for early-stage cutaneous T-cell lymphoma. *Arch. Dermatol.* 128, 931, 1992.
17. Hofer, A. et al. Narrowband (311-nm) UV-B therapy for small plaque parapsoriasis and early-stage mycosis fungoides. *Arch. Dermatol.* 135, 1377, 1999.
18. Clark, C. et al. Narrowband TL-01 phototherapy for patch-stage mycosis fungoides. *Arch. Dermatol.* 136, 748, 2000.
19. Gathers, R.C. et al. Narrowband UVB phototherapy for early-stage mycosis fungoides. *J. Am. Acad. Dermatol.* 47, 191, 2002.
20. Plettenberg, H. et al. Ultraviolet A1 (340–400 nm) phototherapy for cutaneous T-cell lymphoma. *J. Am. Acad. Dermatol.* 41, 47, 1999.
21. von Kobyletski, G. et al. Ultraviolet-A1 phototherapy improves the status of the skin in cutaneous T-cell lymphoma. *Br. J. Dermatol.* 140, 768, 1999.
22. Stander, H. and Schwartz, T. Ultraviolet A1 (340–400 nm) phototherapy for cutaneous T-cell lymphoma? *J. Am. Acad. Dermatol.* 42, 881, 2000.
23. Zane, C. et al. "High-dose" UVA1 therapy of widespread plaque-type, nodular, and erythrodermic mycosis fungoides. *J. Am. Acad. Dermatol.* 44, 629, 2001.
24. Gilchrest, B.A., Parrish, J.A., and Tanenbaum, L. Oral methoxsalen photochemotherapy of mycosis fungoides. *Cancer* 38, 683, 1976.
25. Stern, R. et al. The risk of melanoma in association with long-term exposure to PUVA. *J. Am. Acad. Dermatol.* 44, 755, 2001.
26. Diedcren, P.V.M.M. et al. Narrowband UVB and psoralen-UVA in the treatment of early-stage mycosis fungoides: A retrospective study. *J. Am. Acad. Dermatol.* 48, 215, 2003.
27. Thomsen, K. et al. Retinoids plus PUVA (RePUVA) and PUVA in mycosis fungoides. A report from the Scandinavian Mycosis Fungoides Group. *Acta Derm. Venereol.* 69, 536, 1989.
28. McGinnis, K.S. et al. Psoralen plus long-wave UV-A and bexarotene therapy. An effective and synergistic combined adjunct to therapy for patients with advanced cutaneous T-cell lymphoma. *Arch. Dermatol.* 139, 771, 2003.
29. Roenigk, H.H., Jr. et al. Photochemotherapy alone or combined with interferon alpha-2a in the treatment of cutaneous T-cell lymphoma. *J. Invest. Dermatol.* 95, 198S, 1990.
30. Mostow, E.N. et al. Complete remissions in psoralen and UV-A (PUVA)-refractory mycosis fungoides-type cutaneous T-cell lymphoma with combined interferon alfa and PUVA. *Arch. Dermatol.* 129, 747, 1993.
31. Duvic, M., Hester, J.P., and Lemak, N.A. Photopheresis therapy for cutaneous T-cell lymphoma. *J. Am. Acad. Dermatol.* 35, 573, 1996.
32. Edelson, R. et al. Treatment of cutaneous T-cell lymphoma by extracorporeal photochemotherapy. Preliminary results. *New England J. Med.* 316, 297, 1987.
33. Russell-Jones, R. Extracorporeal photopheresis in cutaneous T-cell lymphoma. Inconsistent data underline the need for randomized studies. *Br. J. Dermatol.* 142, 16, 2000.
34. Gottlieb, S.L. et al. Treatment of cutaneous T-cell lymphoma with extracorporeal photopheresis monotherapy and in combination with recombinant interferon alfa: a 10-year experience at a single institution. *J. Am. Acad. Dermatol.* 35, 946, 1996.
35. Suchin, K.R. et al. Treatment of cutaneous T-cell lymphoma with combined immunomodulatory therapy: a 14-year experience at a single institution. *Arch. Dermatol.* 138, 1054, 2002.

36. Jones, G.W. et al. Total skin electron radiation in the management of mycosis fungoides: consensus of the European Organization for Research and Treatment of cancer (EORTC) cutaneous lymphoma project group. *J. Am. Acad. Dermatol.* 47, 364, 2002.
37. Wilson, L.D. Delivery and sequelae of total skin electron beam therapy. *Arch. Dermatol.* 139, 812, 2003.
38. Wright, J.C. et al. Observations on the use of cancer chemotherapeutic agents in patients with mycosis fungoides. *Cancer* 17, 1045, 1964.
39. Zackheim, H.S., Kashani-Sabet, M., and Hwang, S.T. Low-dose methotrexate to treat erythrodermic cutaneous T-cell lymphoma: results in twenty-nine patients. *J. Am. Acad. Dermatol.* 34, 626, 1996.
40. Zackheim, H.S., Kashani-Sabet, M., and McMillan, A. Low-dose methotrexate to treat mycosis fungoides: a retrospective study in 69 patients. *J. Am. Acad. Dermatol.* 49, 873, 2003.
41. Olsen, E.A. and Bunn, P.A. Interferon in the treatment of cutaneous T-cell lymphoma. *Hematol./Oncol. Clin. North Am.* 9, 1089, 1995.
42. Jumbou, O. et al. Long-term follow-up in 51 patients with mycosis fungoides and Sezary syndrome treated by interferon-alfa. *Br. J. Dermatol.* 140, 427, 1999.
43. Chiarion-Sileni, V. et al. Phase II trial of interferon-α-2a plus psoralen with ultraviolet light A in patients with cutaneous T-cell lymphoma. *Cancer* 95, 569, 2002.
44. Stadler, R. et al. Prospective randomized multicenter clinical trial on the use of interferon α-2a plus acitretin versus interferon α-2a plus PUVA in patients with cutaneous T-cell lymphoma stages I and II. *Blood* 92, 3578, 1998.
45. Wollina, U. et al. Treatment of stage II cutaneous T-cell lymphoma with interferon alfa-2a and extracorporeal photochemotherapy: a prospective controlled trial. *J. Am. Acad. Dermatol.* 44, 253, 2001.
46. Duvic, M. et al. Phase 2 and 3 clinical trial of oral bexarotene (Targretin capsules) for the treatment of refractory or persistent early-stage cutaneous T-cell lymphoma. *Arch. Dermatol.* 137, 581, 2001.
47. Duvic, M. et al. Bexarotene is effective and safe for treatment of refractory advanced-stage cutaneous T-cell lymphoma: multinational phase II–III trial results. *J. Clin. Oncol.* 19, 2456, 2001.
48. Olsen, E. et al. Pivotal phase III trial of two dose levels of denileukin diftitox for the treatment of cutaneous T-cell lymphoma. *J. Clin. Oncol.* 19, 376, 2001.
49. Rosen, S.T. and Foss, F.M. Chemotherapy for mycosis fungoides and the Sezary syndrome. *Hematol/Oncol Clin. North Am.* 9, 1109, 1995.
50. Sarris, A.H. et al. Trimetrexate in relapsed T-cell lymphoma with skin involvement. *J. Clin. Oncol.* 20, 2876, 2002.
51. Bouwhuis, S.A. et al. Treatment of late-stage Sezary syndrome with 2-chlorodeoxy-adenosine. *Int. J Dermatol.* 41, 352, 2002.
52. Wollina, U., Graefe, T., and Kaatz, M. Pegylated doxorubicin for primary cutaneous lymphoma: a report on ten patients with follow-up. *J. Cancer Res. Clin. Oncol.* 127, 128, 2001.
53. Wollina, U. et al. Liposomal daunorubicin in tumor stage cutaneous T-cell lymphoma: report of three cases. *J. Cancer Res. Clin. Oncol.* 129, 65, 2003.
54. Zinzani, P.L. et al. Gemcitabine treatment in pretreated cutaneous T-cell lymphoma: experience in 44 patients. *J. Clin. Oncol.* 18, 2603, 2000.
55. Argiris, A. et al. Phase II trial of 9-aminocamptothecin as a 72-h infusion in cutaneous T-cell lymphoma. *Invest. New Drugs* 19, 321, 2001.

56. Fierro, M.T. et al. Combination of etoposide, idarubicin, cyclophosphamide, vincristine, prednisone and bleomycin (VICOP-B) in the treatment of advanced cutaneous T-cell lymphoma. *Dermatol.* 194, 268, 1997.

57. Scarisbrick, J.J. et al. A trial of fludarabine and cyclophosphamide combination chemotherapy in the treatment of advanced refractory primary cutaneous T-cell lymphoma. *Br. J. Dermatol.* 144, 1010, 2001.

58. Lundin, J. et al. Phase 2 study of alemtuzumab (anti-CD52 monoclonal antibody) in patients with advanced mycosis fungoides/Sezary syndrome. *Blood* 101, 4267, 2003.

59. Guitart, J. et al. Long-term remission after allogeneic hematopoietic stem cell transplantation for refractory cutaneous T-cell lymphoma. *Arch. Dermatol.* 138, 1359, 2002.

60. Soligo, D. et al. Treatment of advanced mycosis fungoides by allogeneic stem-cell transplantation with a nonmyeloablative regimen. *Bone Marrow Transplant* 31, 663, 2003.

61. Russell-Jones, R. et al. Autologous peripheral blood stem cell transplantation in tumor-stage mycosis fungoides: predictors of disease-free survival. *Ann. N.Y. Acad. Sci.* 941, 147, 2001.

62. Kuzel, T.M., Junghans, R., and Foss, F.M. Novel agents for cutaneous T-cell lymphoma. *Hematol./Oncol. Clin. North Am.* 17, 1459, 2003.

11 Staging and Prognosis of Cutaneous T-Cell Lymphoma

*Mohammed Kashani-Sabet and
Herschel S. Zackheim*

CONTENTS

11.1 INTRODUCTION

Analysis of prognostic factors is an important exercise for any malignancy in order to develop staging classifications, stratification factors for clinical trials, and treatment algorithms. Moreover, understanding of the crucial prognostic factors that drive the progression of any cancer is important to understand the biology of that malignancy as it pertains to patient care and education. A staging classification is a crucial instrument for communication between investigators and centers and should describe the important pathways of progression for that malignancy. In this chapter, we undertake a review of advances in our understanding of the various prognostic factors for cutaneous T-cell lymphoma (CTCL), including clinical, histopathological, and molecular factors that help describe the outcome associated with this disease. Moreover, we discuss the current staging classification for CTCL and attempts to revise the staging classification using the advances in prognostic factor identification and analysis.

11.2 PROGNOSTIC FACTORS FOR CTCL

CTCL is a disease entity with a heterogeneous clinical presentation that encompasses two separate forms of cutaneous lymphoma: mycosis fungoides (MF) and Sezary syndrome. Thus, analysis of the various prognostic factors analyzed and described for this disorder is of utmost importance in understanding the factors that are truly important to consider in caring for patients with this multifaceted disorder. We have broadly defined prognostic factors using three categories — namely, clinical factors, histopathological factors, and blood markers — and we review the data for each category of factors to help the reader gain a better understanding of the factors that cause or are associated with disease progression in CTCL.

11.2.1 CLINICAL PROGNOSTIC FACTORS

Several clinical (or demographic) prognostic factors have been examined for their importance in CTCL. These include gender, race, age, and clinical staging, primarily consisting of extent of body surface area (BSA) involvement and clinical presentation — namely, patches and plaques versus tumors versus erythroderma. In this section, we review primarily the demographic factors for their prognostic role in CTCL, as well as extent of skin involvement. The importance of prognostic factors included in the staging classification is discussed in the staging section of the chapter.

A number of studies have examined the role of gender, race, and age in the outcome associated with CTCL. With respect to gender and race, single-institution retrospective studies have failed to demonstrate a significant association between these factors and overall or disease-specific survival associated with CTCL, perhaps due to small sample sizes of certain racial groups. However, a population-based study using the Surveillance, Epidemiology and End Results (SEER) database by Weinstock and Reynes indicated a worse outcome for black patients both in univariate and in multivariate analysis.[1] However, this analysis did not include clinical information such as skin involvement and clinical staging. Therefore, it is unclear whether older or black patients would have a more advanced stage at initial presentation that may account for their worsened survival, as suggested by a study performed by Zackheim and colleagues.[2] In two single-institution studies, age was adversely associated with survival by multivariate analysis.[3,4] However, the breakpoints to define advanced age have differed greatly, from 57 years of age[3] to 75 years of age.[1] Moreover, older patients have been shown to present with more advanced disease.[2,3] Therefore, the independent prognostic impact of age is still unclear. There is a need for confirmation of these observations in other studies that use disease-specific survival or relative survival and compare subjects with an otherwise matched patient population.

11.2.2 HISTOLOGIC PROGNOSTIC FACTORS

Numerous histologic parameters have been evaluated for their prognostic impact in CTCL. In this section, we focus primarily on those factors that have been rigorously evaluated in studies with a large number of patients. Attempts to develop or examine burden or on histological features that portend a poorer outcome. In this section, we thus discuss three pathological markers: tumor burden, as determined by depth of cutaneous infiltrate, large cell transformation, and follicular involvement by MF.

With respect to tumor burden, in 1876 Bazin[5] described the currently accepted model of tumor progression in classical MF, beginning with patch stage and progressing to plaque and tumor stages. However, the exact definition of these stages has remained controversial and has differed between different investigators and centers. In fact, to date, there is no consensus regarding the definitions of patch or plaque-stage disease and whether clinical or histological criteria (or both) should be used in their definition.

Despite this controversy, in 1979, Sanchez and Ackerman[6] described histologic criteria for patch-stage MF. Patch-stage disease was characterized by slight psoriasiform epidermal hyperplasia, a fibrotic papillary dermis, and a sparse papillary dermal and intraepidermal lymphocytic infiltrate. Clinically, these lesions are characterized by erythematous patches with fine scale (except in the case of hypopigmented MF), usually devoid of infiltration or induration. More recently, histologic criteria for plaque-stage MF have been proposed to include similar architectural features as seen in patch-stage MF, but with a more dense lichenoid infiltrate, which also involves the reticular dermis, and conspicuous cellular atypia.[7] Clinically, plaque-stage MF typically presents as erythematous plaques with more extensive scales and would encompass lesions with infiltration or induration. However, there is not perfect agreement between histologic and clinical presentations of patch and plaque-stage disease,[8] prompting some investigators to use a combination of clinical and histologic features.

Nevertheless, recent studies have clearly indicated that the survival of patients presenting with histologically defined patch-stage MF, regardless of extent of body surface area involvement, is unaffected when compared with a matched population.[2] With a trend toward diagnosing CTCL at earlier points in tumor progression,[2] these criteria allow the identification of a patient population with a potentially benign clinical course that obviates the need for aggressive or toxic systemic treatment regimens.[1,9] Similarly, Marti and colleagues have examined the prognostic utility of a "Breslow's thickness" model of depth of lymphomatous infiltrate. Their studies have suggested that lesions thicker than 1 mm (measured from the granular layer to the lower limit of the infiltrate) have a worse prognosis when analyzed by multivariate analysis.[10]

Finally, a recent study by Burg and colleagues attempted to describe a mathematical model to calculate the total tumor burden index in a given patient with MF depending on the presence of various types of infiltrate when defined clinically.[11] Thus, the tumor burden index was calculated by the following formula: (patches $\times$ 2) + (plaques $\times$ 2) + (tumor $\times$ 1.3). Analysis of the tumor burden index in 116 patients suggested that it was a better predictor of survival than the tumor node metastasis (TNM) stage.

In conclusion, while further discussion is required in order to develop consensus regarding the exact criteria used to define the depth of the infiltrate in MF, the prognostic value of this measure is becoming increasingly clear. Moreover, from a staging standpoint, the use of prognostic criteria that describe and conform to the

Distinct from the depth of the cutaneous infiltrate, two other histological criteria that have been evaluated for their prognostic impact and that deserve mention here include large cell transformation and folliculotropic involvement by MF. Large cell transformation has recently been defined as the presence of large cells ($\geq$ 4 times the size of a small lymphocyte in more than 25% of the infiltrate) or the presence of microscopic nodules.[12] Using these criteria, 26 patients out of a database of 115 patients with CTCL were found to have large cell transformation, resulting in a 39% actuarial cumulative probability of transformation in 12 years. Transformation was especially common (46% frequency) in tumor-stage disease. The median survival of the transformed group was significantly lower both from the time of initial diagnosis and from the time of transformation. In addition, patients in whom transformation occurred within 2 years of the initial diagnosis or was accompanied by more advanced stages (tumor or above) had an especially poor prognosis.[12] However, large cell transformation was not an independent predictor of outcome associated with CTCL when analyzed by multivariate analysis.[12] Another study of 45 transformed cases found a similar prognosis for transformed MF and for pleomorphic large T-cell CD30-negative lymphoma.[13]

Finally, a recent study has suggested that follicular MF is a distinct entity that may need to be differentiated from classical MF from a prognostic and potentially even therapeutic standpoint.[14] In this study, 51 patients with follicular MF (49 with associated follicular mucinosis and 2 without) were followed, and their outcome was compared to that of 122 patients with plaque- or tumor-stage MF. Clinical characteristics that distinguished follicular from classical MF included a predilection for involvement of the head and neck and the presence of follicular papules, alopecia, and acneiform lesions. The actuarial 5-year disease-specific survival was 68%, and 10-year survival was 26%. Thus, the survival of follicular MF was worse than that of plaque-stage MF, thereby more closely resembling that of tumor-stage disease. Moreover, follicular MF appeared to be more difficult to treat, with fewer complete responders to various therapies and a higher rate of disease progression. It will be important to analyze follicular MF in the context of classical disease by entering it as a covariate in a Cox regression model in order to accept it as a distinct prognostic entity.

11.2.3 Significance of Blood Involvement in CTCL

11.2.3.1 Prognostic Factors in Erythrodermic CTCL

Given its distinct clinical presentation from MF, a number of studies have examined the role of prognostic factors for erythrodermic CTCL. With respect to clinical factors, younger age (< 65 years of age) was associated with an improved prognosis in one study,[15] but this was not corroborated in others.[16,17] Two important factors that have been analyzed for their prognostic significance include presence of lymph node involvement and peripheral blood involvement. Lymph node involvement (thus upstaging patients to stage IVA) has been shown to be of prognostic significance in a few studies[15,17] when analyzed by Cox regression analysis. By contrast, presence of palpable lymphadenopathy alone was not associated with a worse prognosis.[15]

Blood involvement in erythrodermic CTCL has been analyzed using different methodology: number of circulating Sezary cells (with breakpoints of >5% to >20%) and presence of T-cell clone by Southern blot or polymerase chain reaction (PCR). Patients with more than 5% circulating Sezary cells in the peripheral blood were shown in one study to have a worse prognosis that persisted upon multivariate analysis.[15] However, in another study, Sezary cell count of more than 20% was not independently predictive of survival in erythrodermic CTCL when serum interleukin-2 receptor (sIL-2R) levels were also included in the model (see the next section).[18]

One study that examined the significance of clonal T-cell rearrangements by PCR[17] found hematologic stage to be an important indicator of survival in univariate but not multivariate analysis. However, likelihood ratio tests were utilized to demonstrate that presence of a T-cell clone in the peripheral blood provided additional prognostic information in patients with a defined nodal stage.

Finally, in a study of 62 Sezary patients, several variables were evaluated for their prognostic significance that have not been examined in many other studies.[16] Univariate analysis revealed prior history of MF, high number of circulating leukocytes, Sezary cells, and CD4+ cells, presence of large circulating Sezary cells, elevated serum lactate dehydrogenase (LDH) levels, presence of PAS-positive inclusions in the cytoplasm in circulating Sezary cells, high CD4/CD8 ratio, and CD7-negative circulating Sezary cells to be important predictors of survival. However, only PAS-positive cytoplasmic inclusions, CD7-negativity, and presence of large circulating Sezary cells emerged as independent prognostic factors in stepwise multivariate analysis. Importantly, this study did not include lymph node status, which as previously indicated is the dominant prognostic factor in a number of analyses. In general, analysis of prognostic factors in Sezary syndrome is confounded by small samples sizes and the different criteria or techniques utilized to indicate the presence of blood involvement. Thus, while it is likely that lymph node and blood involvement represent important prognostic factors in the setting of erythrodermic disease, further studies are required to define the precise role of these and other putative factors.

11.2.3.2 Significance of Serum Markers in CTCL

Given that CTCL is a systemic disease with skin-homing characteristics in its early stages, the advent of a serum marker that would accurately reflect tumor burden independently of extent of skin disease would represent a significant advance in the prognostic assessment of CTCL and in the evaluation of response to various therapies. Thus, numerous studies have examined the role of various serum markers for their prognostic significance in CTCL. This discussion will primarily focus on the following factors: IL-2R, LDH, beta-microglobulin, and positive clonal gene rearrangement in the blood.

Wasik et al.[18] evaluated the prognostic role of sIL-2R by enzyme-linked immunosorbent assay in 101 patients with CTCL. Intriguingly, mean sIL-2R levels correlated with skin tumor burden, as they increased in value from patch to plaque to tumor-stage disease. Elevated sIL-2R levels (defined as exceeding 1000 U/mL) were also present in increasing numbers in the progression from patch to tumor-stage MF.

Moreover, sIL-2R levels were correlated with extent of skin involvement, T stage, and LDH levels. However, sIL-2R levels were not independently predictive of survival in CTCL by multivariate analysis in which clinical subtype and T stage emerged as independent covariates. In addition, sIL-2R levels were separately evaluated in the setting of erythrodermic disease. There was no significant difference in sIL-2R levels between patients with erythrodermic MF and those with Sezary syndrome. However, sIL-2R levels were higher in patients with higher Sezary counts (classified as >20%) than those with fewer cells. In univariate analysis, stage and sIL-2R were significantly associated with survival. However, sIL-2R level was the only factor to emerge as an independent factor in multivariate analysis, suggesting its importance as a prognostic factor primarily in the setting of Sezary syndrome.

Second, LDH levels have also been evaluated as a possible prognostic factor in CTCL. Elevated LDH levels were significantly associated with poorer outcome by Cox regression analysis in one study.[4] Other studies have suggested the importance of LDH levels in univariate analysis in the setting of Sezary syndrome[16] or through its association with sIL-2R levels.[18] However, additional studies are required to firmly establish LDH levels as an independent marker of outcome associated with CTCL. Similarly, beta-microglobulin levels were shown to be of prognostic significance in the same study that analyzed the role of LDH levels[4] in univariate but not in multivariate analysis. Thus, the significance of beta-microglobulin levels as a prognostic marker of CTCL is currently uncertain.

Finally, presence of a clone in the peripheral blood has been examined for its prognostic role in CTCL. Fraser-Andrews et al.[19] examined the presence of the T-cell receptor gamma gene in the peripheral blood of 56 patients with CTCL by using the PCR–single strand conformational polymorphism technique. Percent positivity by PCR increased with increasing stage: 21% in T1, 35% in T2, 58% in T3, and 71% in T4. Using Cox regression analysis, peripheral blood clonality provided independent prognostic information after inclusion of age as well as skin and lymph node stage in the model. However, these results have not been corroborated in other studies, perhaps due to sample size or methodological differences. Thus, while it is intriguing to consider the role of several serum factors as a marker of tumor burden and as an independent predictor of survival, further studies are required before any of the aforementioned factors can be routinely used in the evaluation and management of patients with CTCL.

11.3   STAGING OF CTCL

11.3.1   CURRENT STAGING CLASSIFICATION FOR CTCL

Table 11.1 depicts the current staging classification for CTCL that was adopted in 1979 following the recommendations of the Committee on Staging and Classification of Cutaneous T-cell Lymphomas.[20] The T stage stratifies patients on the basis of extent of skin involvement and presence of tumors or erythroderma. Thus, T1 represents patches and plaques involving less than 10% of BSA, while T2 encompasses patients with greater than 10% BSA involvement. Subsequently, T3 disease

TABLE 11.1
Tumor Node Metastasis (TNM) and Staging Classification for Cutaneous T-Cell Lymphoma

T: Skin

    T0: Clinically and/or histopathologically suspicious lesions

    T1: Limited plaques, papules, or eczematous patches covering less than 10% of the skin surface

    T2: Generalized plaques, papules, or erythematous patches covering greater than or equal to 10% of the skin surface

    T3: Tumors (one or more)

    T4: Generalized erythroderma

N: Lymph nodes

    N0: No clinically abnormal peripheral lymph nodes, pathology negative for cutaneous T-cell lymphoma

    N1: Clinically abnormal peripheral lymph nodes, pathology negative for cutaneous T-cell lymphoma

    N2: No clinically abnormal peripheral lymph nodes, pathology positive for cutaneous T-cell lymphoma

    N3: Clinically abnormal peripheral lymph nodes, pathology positive for cutaneous T-cell lymphoma

B: Peripheral blood

    B0: Atypical circulating cells not present (< 5%)

    B1: Atypical circulating cells present (> 5%)

M: Visceral organs

    M0: No visceral organ involvement

    M1: Visceral organ involvement

Staging

IA	T1	N0	M0
IB	T2	N0	M0
IIA	T1,2	N1	M0
IIB	T3	N0,1	M0
III	T4	N0,1	M0
IVA	T1-4	N2,3	M0
IVB	T1-4	N0-3	M1

Source: Bunn, P.A. and Lamberg, S.I. *Cancer Treat. Rep.* 63, 725, 1979.

cation is based on presence of palpable lymphadenopathy and/or evidence of pathologic evaluation of the biopsied lymph node. Thus, N0 disease reveals no palpable lymphadenopathy and no pathologic evidence of CTCL, N1 represents palpable lymphadenopathy without evidence of pathologic involvement, N2 encompasses cases involving blind biopsies of lymph nodes that show evidence of CTCL pathologically, and N3 disease encompasses cases of palpable lymphadenopathy accompanied by pathological evidence of CTCL. The M stage stratifies patients into M0, representing no evidence of visceral organ metastasis, and M1, representing evidence of visceral organ involvement. Finally, given its unique presentation, CTCL staging also has a B (blood) stage to document absence (B0) or presence (B1) of peripheral blood involvement. This was defined at the time to include more than 5% atypical

With respect to staging of CTCL, stage I disease encompasses T1 and T2 cases, divided into stage IA and IB, respectively. Stage IIA comprises N1 cases with palpable lymphadenopathy (but no pathologic involvement). Stage IIB encompasses tumor-stage or T3 disease, whereas stage III represents T4 cases, or erythroderma. Finally, stage IV is divided into IVA, representing nodal metastasis (N2 or 3 disease), and stage IVB, representing all cases with visceral involvement (M1).

11.3.2 ALTERNATIVE STAGING PROPOSALS FOR CTCL

This staging system was introduced on the basis of a survival analysis performed by the Mycosis Fungoides Cooperative Group.[21] A subsequent analysis of the Cooperative Group patients with longer follow up also confirmed the separation in survival between T1–T4 skin stages and between overall stages I–IV.[21] However, this updated analysis also found the number of sites of clinically enlarged lymph nodes to be of prognostic significance and proposed four clinical stages or risk groups on the basis of the T stage and number of clinically enlarged nodal sites. Surprisingly, no changes have been made to the staging of CTCL since the adoption of the 1979 scheme, even though several investigators have probed the utility of various factors in the further refinement of the prognosis associated with CTCL.[22] More recently, Sausville and colleagues proposed three prognostic subgroups on the basis of the type of skin involvement and the presence or absence of blood involvement and/or lymph node involvement in a survival analysis of 152 patients.[23] Thus, patients with plaque-only disease, without lymph node, blood, or visceral involvement, composed the "good-risk" group, with a median survival of more than 12 years. Patients with intermediate risk had a median survival of 5 years and had cutaneous tumors or erythroderma or plaque-stage disease with node or blood involvement but no visceral disease or node effacement. Finally, poor-risk patients, with either visceral involvement or node effacement, had a median survival of 2.5 years. This scheme did not take into account the extent of skin involvement, and it grouped tumors and erythroderma into one clinical stage.

In a recent study, Zackheim et al.[2] analyzed the survival of 489 patients with CTCL seen at a single institution and compared with a matched cohort. Consistent with other available evidence, there was a trend toward earlier diagnosis of CTCL, with a higher percentage of T1 cases and a lower percentage of T3 cases. Moreover, there was no significant difference in survival between patients with T3 and T4 disease, similar to results in several other previous reports.[3,23] When a comparison of relative survival was performed, intriguing observations were made. Stage T1 patients had a similar survival to matched controls, consistent with a previous report of this subgroup.[3] However, the survival of T2 through T4 patients was worse compared with a matched population.[2] In the T2 category though, there were differences in the outcome of patients with T2 patch-stage versus T2 plaque-stage disease.[2] Thus, while the survival of T2 plaque-stage patients was reduced compared with the control population, the survival of T2 patch-stage patients was unaffected. A subsequent analysis also showed that the survival of T2 plaque-stage patients was significantly worse than that of T2 patch-stage patients,[24] further indicating that T2 disease should be stratified by the depth of the infiltrate. A survival analysis that examined all stages of CTCL revealed a significant overlap between survival of stage IB and IIA patients and stage IIB and III patients.

Thus, this analysis indicated that recent definitions of patch-stage MF, along with a trend toward earlier diagnosis of CTCL, have resulted in the identification of a subgroup of patients with a particularly favorable outcome. Given that CTCL has been considered by some authors to be a disease with a uniformly poor prognosis, the identification and stratification of patient subgroups with a better than expected outcome would represent an important goal of a staging classification. This observation has important implications regarding therapy, in that patients with patch-stage disease, regardless of the extent of surface involvement, can be initially treated with more conservative (i.e., skin-directed) treatment modalities, thereby preserving more intensive, toxic, or costly therapies for those patients with a deeper infiltrate or who have progressive disease. Finally, this analysis indicated the similar survival of patients with T3 and T4 disease, suggesting the possibility of grouping T3 and T4 disease for prognostic purposes.[2] While these represent distinct clinical presentations of CTCL, they both represent the final pathway of tumor progression in the skin, whether through the Bazin[5] patch–plaque–tumor model of progression or through the increasing-extent-of-skin-involvement paradigm. Interestingly, several other proposed staging schemes have also suggested combining T3 and T4 into stage III for prognostic purposes.[25,26]

As a result of this analysis, in a subsequent report, Kashani-Sabet et al.[24] examined the utility of an alternative staging scheme for CTCL. This proposal intended to take into account several observations: (1) a trend toward earlier diagnosis of CTCL, (2) the definition of patch-stage MF at the histologic level, (3) the failure of the current staging classification to take into account the patch–plaque–tumor model of CTCL progression, (4) the similar survival of T3 and T4 patients, (5) and the need for the staging classification to define prognostic subgroups that result in a worsening survival with advancing stage.

In the modified staging classification (Table 11.2), a single change was incorporated into the T stage, namely, the splitting of T2 disease into T2a, reflecting patches greater than or equal to 10% BSA, and T2b, reflecting plaques greater than or equal to 10% BSA. T3 and T4 disease still encompassed tumors and erythroderma, respectively, to preserve the distinct clinical presentations. No modifications were made to the B, N, or M stages. In the staging classification, the following changes were made: stage IB would represent T2a (patch-stage) disease greater than or equal to 10% BSA, stage IIB would represent T2b (plaque-stage) disease, stage IIA would not include T2b (plaque-stage) disease, and stage III would encompass both tumor (IIIA) and erythroderma (IIIB). Kaplan–Meier survival plots revealed more even breakpoints between the various proposed new stages, with more natural breakpoints defining stage I, II, and III disease. In this scheme, patients with stage I disease represented a cohort whose survival was unaffected compared with a matched population. Finally, as noted consistently throughout this chapter, multivariate analysis is crucial to examine the independent impact of various prognostic factors. Thus, in this analysis, a Cox regression analysis that included demographic factors and the current and proposed staging classifications, the proposed staging classification

TABLE 11.2

Proposed Tumor Node Metastasis (TNM) and Staging Classification for Cutaneous T-Cell Lymphoma

T: Skin

    T1: Patches and/or plaques covering less than 10% of the skin surface

    T2a: Patches covering greater than or equal to 10% of the skin surface

    T2b: Plaques covering greater than or equal to 10% of the skin surface

    T3: Tumor stage

    T4: Generalized erythroderma (80% or more of skin surface)

N: Lymph nodes

    N0: No clinically abnormal peripheral lymph nodes, pathology negative for cutaneous T-cell
      lymphoma

    N1: Clinically abnormal peripheral lymph nodes, pathology negative for cutaneous T-cell lymphoma

    N2: No clinically abnormal peripheral lymph nodes, pathology positive for cutaneous T-cell
      lymphoma

    N3: Clinically abnormal peripheral lymph nodes, pathology positive for cutaneous T-cell lymphoma

B: Peripheral blood

    B0: Atypical circulating cells not present (<5%)

    B1: Atypical circulating cells present (≥5%)

M: Visceral organs

    M0: No visceral organ involvement

    M1: Visceral organ involvement (confirmed by pathology)

Staging

IA	T1	N0	M0
IB	T2a	N0	M0
IIA	T1,2a	N1	M0
IIB	T2b	N0,1	M0
IIIA	T3	N0,1	M0
IIIB	T4	N0,1	M0
IVA	T1-4	N2,3	M0
IVB	T1-4	N0-3	M1

classification. Thus, the incorporation of two changes (splitting T2 disease into patch and plaque stage and incorporating tumors and erythroderma into stage III) into the staging classification provided a superior measure of CTCL prognosis.

11.4 SUMMARY

In this chapter, we have undertaken a rigorous review of the myriad prognostic factors that have been studied in an attempt to refine the prognostic assessment of patients with CTCL. As indicated, the identification of new prognostic factors is crucial to our attempts to understand the biology of CTCL, to translate this information in a meaningful way to our patients, to stratify patients in clinical trials, and to use as a basis for making treatment decisions. Moreover, modifications and refinements of the staging classification for CTCL over time will allow us to incorporate recent knowledge and concepts into a practical format for discussion with patients and for communication between investigators. In the future, it will be important for larger, multicenter studies of CTCL prognosis to take place in order to develop consensus on crucial definitions of the various proposed prognostic factors and in order to confirm and validate the importance of proposed prognostic staging and prognostic classifications.

REFERENCES

1. Weinstock, M.A. and Reynes, J. F. The changing survival of patients with mycosis fungoides: a population-based assessment of trends in the United States. *Cancer* 85, 208, 1999.
2. Zackheim, H.S. et al. Prognosis in cutaneous T-cell lymphoma by skin stage: long-term survival in 489 patients. *J. Am. Acad. Dermatol.* 40, 418, 1999.
3. Kim, Y.H. et al. Long-term outcome of 525 patients with mycosis fungoides and Sézary syndrome: clinical prognostic factors and risk for disease progression. *Arch. Dermatol.* 139, 857, 2003.
4. Diamandidou, E. et al. Prognostic factor analysis in mycosis fungoides/Sézary syndrome. *J. Am. Acad. Dermatol.*, 40, 914, 1999.
5. Bazin, P.A.E. Maladies de la Peau Observées à l´Hpîtal St. Louis. Paris, 1876.
6. Sanchez, J.L. and Ackerman, A.B. The patch stage of mycosis fungoides: criteria for histologic diagnosis. *Am. J. Dermatopathol.* 1, 5, 1979.
7. LeBoit, P.E. and McCalmont, T.H. Cutaneous lymphomas and leukemias, in *Lever's Histopathology of the Skin*, Elder, D. et al., Eds., Lippincott-Raven, Philadelphia, 1997, chap. 32.
8. Zackheim, H.S., Kashani-Sabet, M., and Amin, S. Topical corticosteroids for mycosis fungoides: experience in 79 patients. *Arch. Dermatol.* 134, 949, 1998.
9. Burg, G. et al. From inflammation to neoplasia: mycosis fungoides evolves from reactive inflammatory conditions (lymphoid infiltrates) transforming into neoplastic plaques and tumors. *Arch. Dermatol.* 137, 949, 2001.
10. Marti, R.M. et al. Prognostic clinicopathologic factors in cutaneous T-cell lymphoma. *Arch. Dermatol.* 127, 1511, 1991.
11. Schmid, M.H. et al. Tumor burden index as a prognostic tool for cutaneous T-cell lymphoma. *Arch. Dermatol.* 135, 1204, 1999.
12. Diamandidou, E. et al. Transformation of mycosis fungoides/Sézary syndrome. *Blood* 92, 1150, 1998.
13. Vergier, B. et al. for the French Study Group on Cutaneous Lymphomas. Transformation of mycosis fungoides: clinicopathological and prognostic features of 45 cases. *Blood* 95, 2212, 2000.
14. Van Doorn, R., Scheffer, E., and Willemze, R. for the Dutch Cutaneous Lymphoma Group. Follicular mycosis fungoides, a distinct disease entity with or without associated follicular mucinosis. *Arch. Dermatol.* 138, 191, 2002.
15. Kim, Y.H. et al. Prognostic factor in erythrodermic mycosis fungoides and the Sézary syndrome, *Arch. Dermatol.* 131, 1003, 1995.
16. Bernengo, M.G. et al. Prognostic factors in Sézary syndrome: a multivariate analysis of clinical, haematological and immunological features. *Ann. Oncol.* 9, 857, 1998.
17. Scarisbrick, J.J. et al. Prognostic significance of tumor burden in the blood of patients with erythrodermic primary cutaneous T-cell lymphoma. *Blood* 97, 624, 2001.

18. Wasik, M.A. et al. Increased serum concentration of the soluble interleukin-2 receptor in cutaneous T-cell lymphoma: clinical and prognostic implications. *Arch. Dermatol.* 132, 42, 1996.
19. Fraser-Andrews, E.A. et al. Detection of a peripheral blood T cell clone is an independent prognostic marker in mycosis fungoides. *J. Invest. Dermatol.* 114, 117, 2000.
20. Bunn, P.A. and Lamberg, S.I. Report of the committee on staging and classification of cutaneous T-cell lymphomas. *Cancer Treat. Rep.*, 63, 725, 1979.
21. Lamberg, S.I. Clinical staging for cutaneous T-cell lymphoma. *Ann. Intern. Med.*, 100, 187, 1984.
22. Foss, F.M. and Sausville, E.A. Prognosis and staging of cutaneous T-cell lymphoma. *Hematol./Oncol. Clin. North Am.* 9, 1011, 1995.
23. Sausville, E.A. et al. Histopathologic staging at initial diagnosis of mycosis fungoides and the Sézary syndrome: definition of three distinctive prognostic groups. *Ann. Intern. Med.* 109, 372, 1988.
24. Kashani-Sabet, M., McMillan, A., and Zackheim, H.S. A modified staging classification for cutaneous T-cell lymphoma. *J. Am. Acad. Dermatol.* 45, 700, 2001.
25. Cohen, S.R. et al. Clinicopathologic relationships, survival, and therapy in 59 patients with observations on occupation as a new prognostic factor. *Cancer* 46, 2654, 1980.
26. Lutzner, M. et al. Cutaneous T-cell lymphomas: the Sézary syndrome, mycosis fungoides, and related disorders. *Ann. Intern. Med.* 83, 534, 1975.

Index